Cognitive Assessment for Clinicians

SECOND EDITION

John R. Hodges

MRC Professor of Behavioural Neurology
University of Cambridge
Department of Clinical Neurosciences
MRC Cognition and Brain Sciences Unit
Cambridge, UK

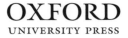

OXFORD
UNIVERSITY PRESS

OXFORD

UNIVERSITY PRESS

Great Clarendon Street, Oxford OX2 6DP

Oxford University Press is a department of the University of Oxford.
It furthers the University's objective of excellence in research, scholarship,
and education by publishing worldwide in

Oxford New York

Auckland Cape Town Dar es Salaam Hong Kong Karachi
Kuala Lumpur Madrid Melbourne Mexico City Nairobi
New Delhi Shanghai Taipei Toronto

With offices in

Argentina Austria Brazil Chile Czech Republic France Greece
Guatemala Hungary Italy Japan Poland Portugal Singapore
South Korea Switzerland Thailand Turkey Ukraine Vietnam

Oxford is a registered trade mark of Oxford University Press
in the UK and in certain other countries

Published in the United States
by Oxford University Press Inc., New York

© Oxford University Press 2007

The moral rights of the author have been asserted
Database right Oxford University Press (maker)

First published 2007

British Library Cataloguing in Publication Data

Data available

Library of Congress Cataloging-in-Publication Data

Hodges, John R.
  Cognitive assessment for clinicians / John R. Hodges. -- 2nd ed.
    p. ; cm.
  Includes bibliographical references and index.
  ISBN 978-0-19-262976-0 (alk.paper)
  1. Cognition -- Testing. 2. Neuropsychological tests. 3. Dementia -- Diagnosis.
  I. Title. [DNLM: 1. Cognition Disorders -- diagnosis. 2. Delirium -- diagnosis.
  3. Dementia -- diagnosis. WM 204 H688c 2007]
  BF311.H6338 2007
  616.8'0475 -- dc22   2007009394

Typeset by Cepha Imaging Private Ltd., Bangalore, India
Printed in Great Britain
on acid-free paper by
CPI Antony Rowe, Chippenham, Wiltshire

ISBN 978–0–19–262976–0

10 9 8 7 6

I dedicate this book to
Adam, Will, and Naomi

Contents

Preface to The First Edition

This book grew out of my experience over the past few years of teaching trainee physicians, psychiatrists, and psychologists about cognitive function and its assessment. I had initially intended to write a very brief pocket guide dealing only with bedside testing. But it became apparent that there was little value in merely describing how to assess cognition, unless the reader had some conceptual knowledge about normal psychological function on which to base the assessment and, most importantly, to guide the interpretation of the examination's findings. The book, therefore, expanded in scope and in size. It now attempts to provide a rational and theoretical basis for cognitive assessment at the bedside or in the clinic, as well as practical guidance on how to take an appropriate history and how to examine patients presenting with disorders of higher cerebral function. The approach advocated in the book is illustrated by twelve case histories of patients seen by me over the last two years. The final section consists of an appendix describing commonly used neuropsychological tests.

When writing the theoretical sections which underpin the assessment, I have drawn on two major strands of research—the traditional localizationalist approach, and the more recent cognitive neuropsychological approach. Most clinicians will be aware of the former; ever since the original observations of Broca, Wernicke, Pick, Dejerine and others in the last century, neurologists have been interested in the cerebral localization of higher mental functions. After a period of relative neglect, recent advances in static (CT and MRI) and functional (PET and SPECT) neuroimaging have reactivated this traditional approach, and considerable advances have been made in the localization of various cognitive functions, which I have attempted to summarize.

The other major strand, cognitive neuropsychology, will be less familiar to clinicians. Most medical curricula still contain only a rudimentary grounding in psychology, and virtually no cognitive neuropsychology. Even some psychology graduates have little experience of this area. Yet in the past two decades there has been an explosion of interest in this field which has produced unparalleled insights into the workings of the human mind. Much of this research originated in Britain, beginning with the pioneering work of John Marshall and Freda Newcombe, and of Elizabeth Warrington and her colleagues. Their experimentally based approach to dissecting the individual subprocesses underlying functions such as reading, object recognition, etc., paved the way for working out the detailed cognitive models that now exist and can be tested experimentally. These and kindred researchers have stressed the critical importance of single-case studies, and of designing tests which isolate specific and dissociable cognitive processes. I have attempted to introduce readers to this exciting area, and to provide a review of the clinically important advances that have been made in cognitive neuropsychology.

Unfortunately, the two major research traditions have, until recently, carried on independently, so that although we now know a great deal about the cognitive basis of many aspects of language, memory, and perception, the neural bases of these processes remain largely unknown. This creates problems when trying to unite these disparate approaches to neuropsychology. In places, the marriage that I have imposed between neurology and cognitive neuropsychology appears rather shaky. It is to be hoped that further advances in the next few years will consolidate our understanding in these areas.

The structure of the book is as follows. Chapters 1 and 2 deal with the theoretical aspects of cognitive function, divided into those which have a widely distributed neural basis (attention/concentration, memory, and highest-order 'executive' function), and those functions which are lateralized to one hemisphere, and often one region of one hemisphere (language, praxis, visuospatial and -perceptual abilities, etc.). Each section of these chapters deals with the neuropsychology, the basic applied anatomy, the clinical disorders, and appropriate tests. The tests mentioned are described in more detail in the Appendix. At the end of Chapter 1 there is also a brief section on delirium and dementia, which constitute the commonest presenting disorders in behavioural neurology and old age psychiatry.

Chapter 3 describes how to take a cognitive history, with a few tips on physical examination. Chapter 4 outlines my approach to assessment at the bedside or in the clinic, and follows the same format as the earlier introductory theoretical chapters. Chapter 5 contains twelve case histories, most of which are taken from our joint neurology–psychiatry cognitive disorders clinic and which illustrate the approach advocated in the earlier chapters. In Chapter 6, I describe the standardized mental test batteries in common use [for example the Mini Mental State Examination, the Blessed Information–Memory–Concentration (IMC) Test, the Hodkinson Brief Mental Test, the Dementia Rating Scale, and the Cambridge Cognitive Examination (CAMCOG)] with notes on their use and abuse. Finally, the Appendix contains details on a selection of neuropsychological tests, consisting of those widely used in neuropsychological practice, with which clinicians should be familiar, and tests which can be given fairly readily by clinicians without specialist training.

I should point out that this is not intended to be a textbook of neuropsychology, of which there are several excellent examples listed under 'Selected

Further Reading' at the end of the book. Neither is it a compendium of neuropsychological tests. It is aimed at clinicians with a nascent, but underdeveloped, interest in cognitive function. The approach advocated forms no substitute for professional psychological evaluation. However, many neurologists and psychiatrists work without adequate neuropsychological provision. By becoming more conversant with bedside cognitive testing, clinicians should be able to use the services of their neuropsychologists more effectively. It is not necessary, for instance, to refer every patient with suspected dementia; many patients can be satisfactorily diagnosed by clinicians if the basic principles outlined in the book are followed. There are, however, patients in whom a thorough neuropsychological evaluation is mandatory, as is illustrated by several of the cases in Chapter 5.

If this book stimulates any trainee neurologist or psychiatrist to develop a special interest in neuropsychology, or to pursue a research career in this field, then it will have more than fulfilled its original aims.

Preface to The Second Edition

The revision of my 'little red book', as it has become affectionately known, has taken far longer than I intended. Within a few years of the publication of the first edition it was clear that a revision was required. I had planned to work on it during my sabbatical year (2002) spent in the glorious city of Sydney, but for mysterious reasons other temptations prevented me from getting down to it. The prospect seemed too daunting, as so many new tasks have been introduced into clinical neuropsychology. In addition, I wanted to incorporate a revision of the formalized bedside test developed in Cambridge, the Addenbrooke's Cognitive Examination (ACE), which has proven so useful in our memory and dementia clinics. By 2004 a revision of the ACE, the ACE-R, was completed which, at last, galvanized me into action. Rather than simply update the book with a few new tests and case vignettes, I have taken the opportunity to radically overhaul the text. In preparing this second edition I have been surprised that the basic principles which guided the first edition still hold up to scrutiny but a lot of changes have been necessary to the content of each chapter. Instead of incorporating delirium and dementia into the first chapter these have been given their own chapter and the whole of the first, theoretical section (Chapters 1–3) has been revised to incorporate new discoveries, ideas, and even a few novel disorders. Chapters 3 and 4 have changed the least but have been updated to reflect my experience of bedside cognitive evaluation over the past decade. The section on standard mental test schedules has been split so that the ACE-R now gets its own chapter (Chapter 7) with a description of uses and limitations together with normative data. The number of illustrative cases has been expanded (Chapter 8) and their description built around the use of the ACE-R in clinical practice. The Appendix required the most revision to reflect the explosion in the number of neuropsychological tests available. I have attempted to describe those in widespread usage but the selection is obviously biased towards tests regularly used in Cambridge.

Acknowledgements

I would like first, and foremost, to acknowledge the intellectual debt I owe to a number of teachers and colleagues who have encouraged my interest in cognitive dysfunction over two decades. Whilst in Oxford, I was fortunate to work with John and Susan Oxbury, who provided an environment in which an interest in neuropsychology was encouraged. The presence of John Marshall and Freda Newcombe in the University Department of Neurology was also a seminal influence. This milieu, which was sadly unique in British neurology at the time, also nurtured the interests of my friends and contemporaries Christopher Ward and Harvey Sagar. At that time I also began a fruitful collaboration with Elaine Funnell, who was working at Birkbeck College. Charles Warlow did much to help by co-supervising my MD project on transient global amnesia when he was Clinical Reader in Oxford, and by implanting the idea of this book on a subsequent visit to Edinburgh.

The Medical Research Council kindly sponsored a fellowship year spent studying neuropsychology at the Alzheimer Disease Research Center in the University of California, San Diego. Whilst I was there, Nelson Butters and David Salmon were particularly influential. It was this year, more than any other, that decided the direction of my future research interests. Nelson, who sadly died of motor neuron disease a few years after my fellowship year, was an inspiration and provided honorary membership of the North American neuropsychology community.

Since moving to Cambridge, I have been extremely fortunate to work closely with a group of outstanding clinical and experimental neuropsychologists. Karalyn Patterson has been a particularly important guiding light, and together we established an active research programme investigating aspects of language and memory in patients with Alzheimer's disease and the frontotemporal dementias which has been going strong for 15 years. Kim Graham graduated from being our first PhD student to postdoctoral fellow and is now a senior scientist and joint co-ordinator of the group based at the MRC Cognition and Brain Sciences Unit (CBU). Over the years, I have also benefited enormously from collaborations with Alan Baddeley, German Berrios, Roz McCarthy, Trevor Robbins, Barbara Sahakian, Ian Robertson and Barbara Wilson. John Xuereb started my neuropathology education which was continued in the beautiful city of Sydney by Glenda Halliday and Jillian Kril. I have been blessed by having a succession of excellent clinical research fellows, many of whom have moved to clinical and academic positions around the world including John Greene, Tom Esmonde, Peter Garrard, Richard Perry, Adam Zeman, Tom Bak, Cath Mummery, Clare Galton, Siân Thompson, Shibley Rahman, Peter Nestor, Rhys Davies, Andrew Graham, Chris Kipps, Jonathan Knibb, Paul McMonagle and George Pengas. We have also benefited from the overseas visitors who have contributed to the research effort, notably Pavagada Mathuranath, Ellajosyula Ratnavalli, Suvarna Alladi, Facundo Manes, Joseph Spatt, Manabu Ikeda and Adrian Ivanoiu. Tim Rogers, Matt Lambon-Ralph, Sasha Bozeat, Anna Adlam and Naida Graham have all been long-term colleagues at the MRC unit.

The memory clinic was founded in 1990 with German Berrios and has provided the basic fuel—a plentiful supply of patients with cognitive disorders for our studies. Our first clinical neuropsychologist, Kristin Breen, sadly passed away at a tragically young age. Since then we have had the pleasure of working with Diana Caine, Aidan Jones and currently Narinder Kapur. Jerry Brown moved to Cambridge a decade ago and has added a valuable genetic dimension to the clinic. The increasing number of patients under follow-up during the 1990s persuaded us to clone the concept of a multidisciplinary cognitive clinic and in 1997 we started an Early Onset Dementia Clinic, largely for follow-up of patients with FTD and their carers. Sinclair Lough brought expertise in clinical psychology to this clinic and, after his move to Dorset, we were fortunate in persuading Vanessa Garfoot to participate in the clinic. Tom Bak deserves special thanks for being such an inspiring colleague and shouldering the burden of the Disorders of Movement and Cognition Clinic for 10 years. At the hospital Kate Dawson has been a tower of strength and support to our patients and their families (together with Angela O'Sullivan and Lynne MacDonald) who have helped so much with the research. Sharon Davies has co-ordinated the research at the MRC-CBU and also used her copy-editing skills in preparing this revision of the book. Margaret Tillson has provided first-rate secretarial skills and tolerated many re-draftings of this book.

J. R. H.
Cambridge
July 2006

Chapter 1

Distributed Cognitive Functions

A General Theoretical Framework

When approaching cognitive assessment patients in the clinic or at the bedside it is essential to have a general structure on which to base the clinical interview and examination. The schema suggested here adopts the general neurological approach of localization followed by differential diagnosis. I have attempted to link anatomy with cognitive function, wherever possible, although the strict localization of many aspects of cognition is still far from clear. Recent functional imaging studies in normal subjects show that virtually all aspects of cognition depend upon the integrated activity of several brain regions. In a quest for clarity and brevity, I have been forced to take a simplified and often didactic approach that necessarily avoids many interesting issues and controversies in neuropsychology and behavioural neuroscience. For those wishing to read more detailed analyses of brain structure–function relationships, and of cognitive neuropsychology in general, several reference sources are suggested in 'Selected further reading' at the end of this book. Thankfully a number of excellent textbooks have been published in the last few years.

The basic dichotomy offered here is between distributed and localized functions. The label *distributed* implies cognitive abilities, which are not strictly localized to one lateralized brain region, as outlined in Table 1.1. Hence abnormalities of these distributed functions do not, with a few notable exceptions (such as amnesia following thalamic strokes), arise from small discrete lesions, but typically result from fairly extensive and often bilateral damage or more generalized insults of the type encountered in general medical practice. *Localized* functions can, in turn, be divided into those associated with the dominant, usually left, hemisphere, and those associated with the non-dominant hemisphere.

In this chapter, I shall describe three broad domains of cognition that have a distributed neural basis: arousal/attention, memory and executive function. Chapter 2 deals with the syndromes of delirium and dementia and Chapter 3 covers localized cognitive abilities. The tests mentioned in Chapters 1, 2 and 3 will be described more fully in subsequent chapters.

Table 1.1 Distributed cognitive functions

Cognitive function	Neural basis
1. Attention/concentration	Reticular activating system (brain stem and thalamic nuclei), and multimodal association areas (prefrontal and parietal) with right bias
2. Memory	Limbic system (especially hippocampus and diencephalon)
3. Higher-order executive functions and social cognition	Frontal lobes

Arousal and Attention

Although attention to the external environments and to our own internal thought processes, is clearly extremely important it remains difficult to state the specific defining characteristics of attention. We all know what to be attentive means in ecological terms, but cognitively attention is a complex ability. During wakefulness an individual is bombarded with a plethora of sensory stimuli originating from the environment arriving via all of our sensory organs. In addition, we are also in a state of constant rumination with thoughts, ideas and memories, which pop into mind, often seemingly at random. Despite this we are able to engage in specific goal-directed behaviours ranging from making breakfast, driving to work, chairing a meeting or solving a series of complex problems. Our attentional processes allow us to focus on specific parts of stimulus space and to hold other stimuli at bay, at least temporarily. We are also able to shift our attention and often to engage in two tasks at once.

There have been many attempts to characterize the various subprocesses embraced within the broad rubric of attention. For clinical purposes the following is a useful classification of the components of attention:

1. Arousal, which describes the general state of responsivity and wakefulness.

2. Sustained attention, or vigilance, refers to the capacity to maintain attentional activity over prolonged periods of time.

3. Divided attention involves the ability to respond to more than one task at once.

4. Selective attention is the capacity to highlight, or focus upon, one stimulus while suppressing awareness of competing stimuli.

A good example of the application of these processes is the ability to drive a car while conversing with a passenger under easy driving conditions, which requires both sustained and divided attention, but as soon as a more complex operation, such as merging lanes or overtaking, is required then it is usually necessary to shift attention and to focus on to the operations involved with driving. The four processes described above are all global, or superordinate, aspects of attention, which operate across sensory domains and can be contrasted to domain-specific attentional abilities (see below).

Orientation, concentration, exploration and vigilance are positive aspects of global attentive processes, while distractibility, impersistence, muddledness and confusion reflect impaired attention. Marked impairment of attention is almost always accompanied by disorientation in time and/or place. The clinical syndrome, which exemplifies a breakdown of global attention at processing, is the acute confusional state (sometimes called acute organic psychiatric syndrome or, more simply, delirium). Although other abnormalities are found in delirium, disordered attention is the principal and most consistent disturbance. When severe, consciousness is diminished due to depression of basic arousal processes.

Rather confusingly, the term attention is also used in the context of so-called domain-specific attention. The most well-known aspect of domain-specific attention is attention to space. Breakdown of this ability results in the spatial neglect commonly seen after right hemisphere strokes. Regions in the non-dominant hemisphere, particularly the inferior parietal and prefrontal regions, have a specialized role in spatial attention, which will be discussed further under the heading of neglect (see Chapter 3).

It is important to know that wakefulness or arousal is only one aspect of attention. In states of diminished wakefulness, noxious stimulation is required to provoke a response that is typically stereotyped and non-purposeful. Patients in such a state are described as being drowsy, stuporosed or in coma, depending on the level of arousal deficit. In patients with diminished awareness, further testing of cognition is clearly pointless and scales such as the Glasgow Coma Scale are more appropriate assessment tools.

Applied anatomy

The maintenance of attention depends upon the interaction of two major neural systems: the ascending reticular activating system (ARAS) which exerts so-called 'bottom-up' modulation of cortical regions and a cortical 'top-down' system of regulation involving limbic, parietal, and especially prefrontal cortical regions. In addition to these two domain-independent systems, there are local 'domain-specific' processes operating in specialized cortical regions which modulate responsivity to sounds, tactile stimuli, motion, faces, objects, words and memories. This overall attentional matrix (in the terms of Marsel Mesulam)

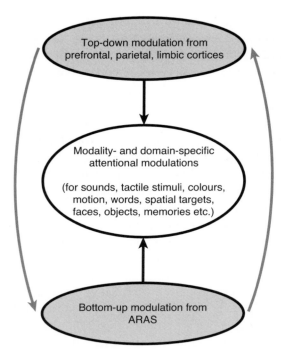

Fig. 1.1 Three compartments of attentional matrix. (Based on work of Marsel Mesulam with permission.)

controls the diverse processes described above (see Figure 1.1). Attention is therefore a collective manifestation of bottom-up, top-down and domain-specific modulation. Disruption of the bottom-up ARAS system produces the syndrome of delirium or, if very severe, coma. Pathology involving the top-down system tends to cause less-pronounced deficits of the type of inattention and distractibility seen following frontal and parietal damage as a result of traumatic brain injury or stroke.

The ARAS contains several components shown in Figure 1.2. Perhaps the best known is the reticulothalamic cortical pathway, which promotes and maintains cortical arousal by facilitating the transthalamic passage of sensory information towards the cortex. Acetylcholine is the major neurotransmitter in the lower, reticulothalamic component of this pathway, while excitatory amino acids (such as glutamate) are important thalamic–cortical transmitters. Other important components of the ARAS are transmitter-specific pathways originating in the brain stem or basal forebrain and projecting to the cerebral cortex. These brain stem components include the dopaminergic projections from the raphe nucleus and the noradrenergic projections from the locus coeruleus. The basal forebrain component includes the cholinergic and

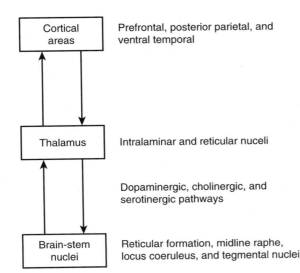

| Cortical areas | Prefrontal, posterior parietal, and ventral temporal |

| Thalamus | Intralaminar and reticular nuceli |

Dopaminergic, cholinergic, and serotinergic pathways

| Brain-stem nuclei | Reticular formation, midline raphe, locus coeruleus, and tegmental nuclei |

Fig. 1.2 Ascending reticular activating system (ARAS): major structures and pathways involved in normal attentional process.

gabanergic pathways originating in the nucleus basalis. Bottom-up modulation of attention depends therefore upon a delicate balance of brain chemical systems. It is not surprising that diverse metabolic abnormalities produce delirium. It should be recalled also that many of these systems are involved in neurodegenerative disorders, which helps to explain the inattentiveness that occurs from an early stage in Parkinson's disease and related syndromes, Alzheimer's disease and particularly in dementia with Lewy bodies.

The posterior parietal, limbic and prefrontal cortices mediate top-down modulation of attention. The parietal cortex is particularly active during functional imaging studies in normal subjects engaged in tests of sustained and selective attention while the dorsolateral prefrontal cortex has a key role in divided attention. Within the limbic system, the anterior cingulate cortex plays a pivotal role in attention, as demonstrated by a series of functional imaging studies in normal subjects. Damage to this region, following bilateral anterior cerebral artery occlusion, or in association with butterfly glioma, produces a state of severe inattentiveness referred to as akinetic mutism.

The thalamus acts as a major relay station between the cortex and the ARAS. The intralaminar nuclei receive inputs from brain stem nuclei and relay information widely to the cortex. A reciprocal feedback loop from the cortex modulates these ascending pathways via the thalamus.

It can be seen from this brief description that global disorders of attention can arise from diverse pathologies involving these bottom-up and top-down modulatory systems. This disruption may result from structural damage or, more commonly, metabolic disorders and pharmacological agents, as described more fully later. Lesser degrees of attentional impairment involve specific components such as selective sustained or divided attention. For instance, impairment in selective attention appears to be particularly common in the early stages of Alzheimer's disease, although such patients also go on to develop divided attention deficits. In dementia with Lewy bodies there is profound impairment of attentional processing and patients with vascular dementias likewise have marked problems with attentional modulation.

Tests of attention

1. Orientation in time and place (also dependent upon episodic memory).
2. Digit span, especially digits backwards.
3. Recitation of the months of the year or days of the week in reverse order or serial subtraction of 7s.
4. Alternation tasks, such as Trails B.
5. Tests of sustained attention such as the Paced Auditory Serial Addition Test (PASAT).
6. The Stroop Test of response inhibition.
7. Timed tests involving letter or star cancellation.
8. Digit-symbol or symbol-digit substitution tests.
9. Components of the Test of Everyday Attention (TEA).

Memory

Introduction

Neuropsychological research in humans with focal brain lesions and in non-human primates following surgical lesions has shown that memory is not a single all-encompassing system. Unfortunately, a plethora of terms has arisen to describe the various subcomponents of memory. One broad distinction divides memory into that available to conscious access and reflection (called **explicit** or **declarative memory**), and those types of learned responses, such as conditioned reflexes, motor skill acquisition and priming which are not available for conscious reflection (called **implicit** or **procedural memory**). Explicit memory is further divided into two systems: one is responsible for the laying down and recall of personally experienced and temporally specific events or episodes called **episodic memory**. The other type of explicit memory is responsible for our permanent store of representational knowledge of facts and concepts, objects and people, as well as words and their meaning, and is termed **semantic memory**. Although in linguistics and philosophy

Table 1.2 Divisions within long-term memory

	Type of material	**Neural substrate**
Explicit		
Episodic	Personally experienced episodes and events; time- and context-specific	Extended limbic system and dorsolateral prefrontal cortex
Semantic	Vocabulary, facts, concepts, object and face knowledge; time- and context-specific	Polar and inferior temporal neocortex (with lateralized specialization)
Implicit		
Procedural	Motor skills, e.g. driving, playing golf Priming Classical conditioning	Basal ganglia Cerebral cortex Unknown, cerebellar?

'semantics' refers purely to the study of word meaning, in neuropsychology semantic memory has a wider use and applies to our general store of world knowledge. Semantic memory begins to be acquired early in life and continues to expand throughout our lifetime. It is organized conceptually, without reference to the time and context in which it was acquired. Both episodic and semantic memory are components of our long-term memory systems (see Table 1.2 and Figure 1.3).

To illustrate this dichotomy further, consider the example of recalling the details of a conversation from earlier in the day or a dinner on holiday in Paris

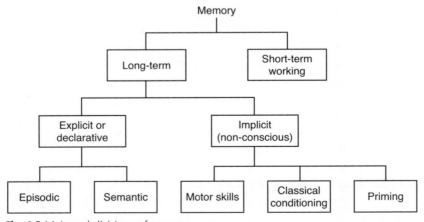

Fig. 1.3 Major subdivisions of memory.

last year, both of which depend upon episodic memory. By contrast, knowing that Paris is the capital of France, what the word 'dinner' means, that a canary is a small yellow bird more closely related to a sparrow than a penguin, and identifying a photograph of Bill Clinton all depend upon our semantic memory. The content of episodic and semantic memory are both available to conscious access. By contrast, the acquisition of motor skills, such as learning to drive a car or play a musical instrument, does not use explicit memory, but instead relies upon the implicit memory system.

The term 'memory disorder' may, therefore, apply to various different types of problem. Most commonly, it is used to mean a disorder of episodic memory, that is to say difficulty recalling personally experienced episodes from the recent past or learning new information. Disorders of episodic memory will be dealt with in more detail below. In brief, they occur either in the context of diffuse brain injury (as part of a dementia), or as a result of selective damage to bilateral limbic structures, when the disorder is pure, spares other aspects of cognition and is termed the 'amnesic syndrome'.

Semantic memory loss is also an integral part of many dementing illnesses, particularly Alzheimer's disease. Isolated impairment of semantic memory is uncommon, but occasionally occurs in the context of anterior temporal lobe damage, particularly in the syndrome of semantic dementia. Profound impairment of episodic and semantic memory occurs in survivors of herpes simplex virus encephalitis.

Short-term (working) memory

In neuropsychological terms, short-term memory is synonymous with the system of working memory responsible for the immediate recall of small amounts of verbal (as in, for example, digit span) or spatial material. It was traditionally held that for new information to enter long-term memory it must first pass through this short-term memory store. Likewise, it was believed that material recalled from long-term memory stores must first be processed by the immediate store. This simplistic serial processing model was rejected following the discovery of brain-injured patients with defective short-term memory but with completely normal ability to lay down and retrieve new longer-term memories. In addition, a number of apparently normal subjects (usually undergraduates who unwisely volunteered for psychology experiments!) have been found to have very limited short-term memory capacity. It is worth noting at this point that patients with very severe deficits in forming new memories, as in Korsakoff's syndrome, have normal short-term memory.

There is now good evidence that there are, in fact, various subcomponents of **working memory** responsible for the immediate repetition of words, numbers, and melodies (called the phonological or articulatory loop) and separately for rehearsal of spatial information (the so-called visuo-spatial or visual sketch pad) both of which are controlled by a system known as the central executive (see Figure 1.4). Working memory appears to function independently of, but in parallel with, longer-term memory. The central executive component of working memory is associated with the dorsolateral prefrontal lobe and is particularly important for dual-task performance, that is to say, when two tests are performed simultaneously. This aspect of working memory is really part of the larger attentional system discussed above.

The phonological loop depends upon peri-sylvian language areas in the dominant (typically left) hemisphere and the visuo-spatial sketch pad is associated with non-dominant parieto-occipital regions. Hence damage to widely dispersed brain regions may impair distinct components of working memory. For example, a reduced digit span is common in aphasic patients with left hemisphere lesions and is also seen in patients with frontal lobe pathology. The mechanisms underlying this deficit are different in these two instances. In the former, the phonological loop system is defective, typically producing a marked reduction in both forward and backward digit span, as well as problems in word and sentence repetition. Span reduction in association with dorsolateral prefrontal lesions is typically more modest involving particularly reverse span and, in contrast to phonological deficits, sparing word and sentence repetition. This is also a common finding in patients with frontal and subcortical dementia syndromes.

Clinicians use the term 'short-term memory' loosely to refer to recall of new material over an ill-defined short period, typically between 5 and 30 min, but sometimes they refer to retention over days or weeks. There is no evidence,

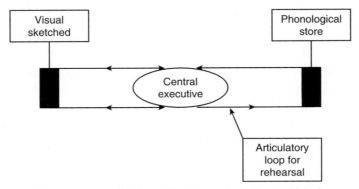

Fig. 1.4 Working memory model. (Based on the work of Alan Baddeley.)

however, either from the study of normal subjects or patients with brain disorders, to support the existence of a storage system with these temporal characteristics. As we have seen above, the neuropsychological evidence points to there being one system that is responsible for very short (or immediate) recall of verbal or spatial material (termed working memory), and a number of longer-term systems responsible for different types of material: episodic, semantic, procedural, etc. This brief discussion highlights the controversy over what is meant by 'short-term memory'. I have therefore avoided discussing short-term memory. When I do apply this term it is used in the neuropsychological sense to refer to immediate or working memory. In clinical practice, a much more useful distinction is between the acquisition of new information (anterograde memory) and the recall of previously learnt material (retrograde memory) since these two components may be impaired independently in different pathologies, as we shall see below.

Tests of working memory

1. Digit span forwards and backwards.
2. Corsi block tapping span.
3. Spatial working memory such as the box search task from the CANTAB battery.
4. Dual performance tests such as simultaneons visual tracking and serial subtraction or digit span.

Episodic memory

Applied anatomy

Extensive studies of patients with acquired focal lesions as well as those who have undergone neurosurgical resections have established which structures are critical for the laying down and retrieval of episodic memories: the medial temporal lobe (particularly the hippocampus, subiculum and the entorhinal cortex); the diencephalon (mamillary bodies, plus the anterior and dorsomedial nuclei of the thalamus with their interconnecting tracts), the basal forebrain nuclei (the septal nucleus, the diagonal band of Broca and the nucleus basalis) and the retrosplenial cortex. All of these structures are bilateral with components in both hemispheres. The principal areas are connected by a number of pathways, including the fornix and the cingulate gyrus. Together these structures constitute the extended limbic system, sometimes referred to as the circuit of Papez (see Figure 1.5). The hippocampus has traditionally been viewed as the core or central component of this system. It receives afferents from, and sends efferents to, each of the higher-order sensory association

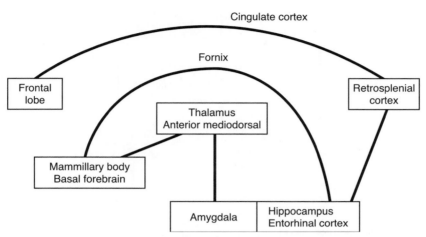

Fig. 1.5 Principal components of the limbic system concerned with episodic memory.

areas (visual, auditory, somatosensory etc.) as well as polysensory areas. The internal circuitry of the hippocampus has been worked out in great detail; inputs arrive at the dentate gyrus via the perforant pathway, which sends efferents back to the association areas and to the mamillary bodies via the fornix; the dentate gyrus projects to CA3 which, in turn, projects to CA1; the latter relays to the subiculum.

Damage anywhere in the limbic system can produce memory deficits but these are often subtle and material-specific. For instance, surgical removal or infarction of the left hippocampus produces a selective memory deficit for verbal material. In contrast, right-sided damage to the same structures produces a specific non-verbal memory problem (for instance, learning new faces or spatial information) which would not be apparent without detailed neuropsychological assessment. Bilateral damage to the medial temporal lobe, the diencephalon or the basal forebrain produces a devastating and profound amnesic syndrome for both verbal and non-verbal material.

There is ongoing debate about specialization within medial temporal lobe structures in terms of recall and recognition memory. There is growing evidence that the hippocampus proper is particularly important for spatial memory and for the recall, as opposed to recognition, of newly learnt material. In addition, it has a special role for cross-modal associative learning: that is to say, learning to associate different types of sensory information such as a pattern with a particular spatial location, or a face with a name.

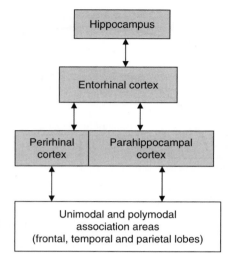

Fig. 1.6 Subregions of the medial temporal lobe.

Recent studies in non-human primates with surgically induced lesions have emphasized the role of the parahippocampal structures, particularly the perirhinal cortex. Lesions to this area cause profound memory impairment affecting both recall and recognition. The relationship between these medial temporal regions is shown in Figure 1.6 and an anatomical illustration is given in Figure 1.7.

Disorders of episodic memory: transient amnesia and the amnesic syndrome

Impaired episodic memory is a feature of both delirium and dementia and in both of these disorders the memory deficit is multifactorial, with contributions

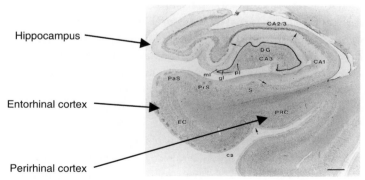

Fig. 1.7 Anatomical cross-section of hippocampus and related parahippocampal structures.

from decreased attention, impaired retrieval strategies, and defective memory *per se*. The term amnesic syndrome should be restricted to patients with pure disorders of memory, sparing other intellectual abilities. Such disorders may be acute and transient, or chronic and generally permanent (see Table 1.3).

Transient amnesia Transient global amnesia (TGA) is an interesting and not uncommon disorder. It typically occurs in later life with a peak around the sixth and seventh decades. Cases under the age of 40 years are exceptional. The apparent tail-off in very late life is probably due to under-reporting. The patient, who is generally in good health, suddenly becomes profoundly amnesic. Short-term (working) memory is preserved, but he or she is unable to retain any new information for more than a few seconds. The profound

Table 1.3 Causes of episodic memory impairment

	Pure amnesia	Mixed (other accompanying cognitive deficits)
Acute (transient)	Transient global amnesia Transient epileptic amnesia Closed head injury Drugs, e.g. benzoadiazapines alcohol Psychogenic (hysterical) fugues	Delirium (see Chapter 2)

Chronic (persistent)	Amnesic syndrome:
	1. *Hippocampal damage*
	   Herpes simplex virus encephalitis
	   Limbic encephalitis (paraneoplastic)
	   Anoxia
	   Surgical removal of temporal lobes
	   Bilateral posterior cerebral artery
	     occlusion
	   Closed head injury
	   Early Alzheimer's disease
	2. *Diencephalic damage*
	   Korsakoff's syndrome
	    (alcoholic and non-alcoholic)
	   IIIrd ventricle tumours and cysts
	   Bilateral thalamic infarction
	   Post-subarachnoid haemorrhage
	    especially from anterior
	    communicating artery
	    aneurysms
	3. *Retrosplenial damage*
	   Tumours
	   Bleeds
	   Alzheimer's disease
		Dementia (see Chapter 2)

anterograde amnesia is accompanied by a variable retrograde memory deficit spreading back weeks, months, or even years. Patients appear disorientated and repetitively ask the same cycle of questions (for example, 'what's happened to me?', 'why am I here?' or 'what day is it?') but there is no impairment of conscious level or attention, and no language or visuo-spatial deficits. After a few hours, typically 4–8, the ability to lay down new memories returns gradually and the retrograde amnesia shrinks so that patients are left with a dense amnesic gap encompassing the duration of the attack, often together with the couple of hours preceding the onset. The rate of recurrence is in the order of 2–3% per year and the general prognosis is excellent. The cause of this syndrome remains unknown but it is clear that thromboembolic cerebrovascular disease does not play a part, at least in the vast majority of cases. There is an association with migraine and with stressful emotional and physical events immediately preceding the attack.

Transient epileptic amnesia (TEA) is a more recently recognized syndrome that resembles TGA. Patients are typically in the same age range as those with TGA although it can occur in younger subjects. Patients present with brief episodes of confusion and disorientation. There is repetitive questioning, as in TGA, but the duration of attacks is generally less than an hour and typically only a few minutes. Attacks often occur immediately upon waking in the morning or after a catnap. Unlike TEA there can be partial recall of the ictus. Episodes are recurrent and may evolve into more typical complex partial seizures. Most patients with TEA also complain of large gaps in their autobiographical memory which come to light when trying to recall the details of holidays or family events undertaken during the past few years. Regular electroencephalogram (EEG) recordings may be normal, but sleep EEGs usually reveal temporal lobe spike or sharp wave activity. The aetiology in many cases seems to be cerebrovascular. Treatment with anticonvulsants typically prevents recurrence of the TEA events but may not improve remote memory loss. Recent studies have shown that patients with TEA have accelerated forgetting of new information; although they perform normally on memory tasks which test recall after 30–60 minutes, patients with TEA show severe impairment when tested after 4 or 6 weeks. It is not clear whether ongoing ictal activity or underlying pathology in the medial temporal lobe causes this 'long-term or accelerated forgetting'.

Acute closed head injury may cause a state very similar to TGA but there is usually very limited retrograde amnesia, and attentional processes are also typically impaired.

Hysterical or psychogenic fugue states are now rare. They occur predominantly in younger adults with a background of psychiatric problems. There is usually a recognizable precipitating life event such as bereavement or impending criminal charges. In contrast to TGA there is a profound retrograde amnesia encompassing the subject's whole life and including loss of personal identity but sometimes without significant anterograde memory impairment.

The amnesic syndrome: defining characteristics

1. Preserved global intellectual abilities. In alcoholic Korsakoff's syndrome frontal executive deficits are frequently present and patients are apathetic but other intellectual abilities are preserved. On neuropsychological testing there should be a significant discrepancy between the general Intelligence Quotient (IQ) and the Memory Quotient (MQ). In patients with medial temporal lobe damage, executive abilities are spared and the amnesia is typically much purer.

2. Anterograde amnesia, i.e. severe impairment of the acquisition of new episodic memories. Patients show impairment on both verbal and non-verbal memory tests. In most instances recall and recognition are impaired although there are reports of patients with pure hippocampal pathology involving particularly recall with relative sparing of recognition.

3. Retrograde amnesia, i.e. impaired recall of past events. The degree of retrograde amnesia depends to some extent on the locus of damage, and hence the aetiology of the amnesic syndrome. Diencephalic amnesia, as exemplified by Korsakoff's syndrome, is characterized by temporally extensive retrograde amnesia covering many decades but with some sparing of more distant memories referred to as a temporal gradient. Hippocampal amnesia, by contrast, may be accompanied by a much shorter retrograde amnesia extending back a couple of years only (see below).

4. Preserved short-term/working memory.

5. Preserved procedural (implicit) memory.

The cognitive neuropsychology of the amnesic syndrome

There is still considerable controversy regarding the basic cognitive deficits underlying the amnesic syndrome. Short-term (working) memory, as judged by digit span or registration of a name and address, is normal. According to contemporary information-processing accounts of memory, the deficit in amnesia could be at any of the following stages:

1. During the initial laying down (encoding) of new memories, perhaps as a result of a defective labeling or tagging;

2. During the process that occurs after initial encoding that is responsible for the consolidation of long-term memory traces; or

3. During the operation of memory retrieval.

Patients with diencephalic amnesia, as in Korsakoff's syndrome, have problems mainly with memory encoding and, hence, lay down weak memory traces. Once information has entered into long-term stores there is little evidence of rapid decay or forgetting. Korsakoff's syndrome patients also have an extensive and temporally graded retrograde amnesia. It has been argued that this remote memory deficit is due to the fact that alcoholics have been encoding weak memories for many years, because they spend their life in an alcohol-induced blur. A number of studies have refuted this suggestion, and it appears that retrieval *per se* is also defective in Korsakoff's syndrome. Moreover, exactly the same picture of severe anterograde and retrograde amnesia can be seen in patients with non-alcohol induced (for example, starvation-induced) Korsakoff's syndrome, and in patients with bilateral thalamic infarction. Hence there seems to be dual pathology, affecting the laying down of new memories, as well as the retrieval of both new and old memories, in diencephalic amnesia.

Hippocampal amnesia, as a result of anoxia or very restricted infarction of medial temporal lobe structures, has been traditionally associated with impaired anterograde amnesia but a temporally limited retrograde amnesia: some patients are said to show deficits in recall of autobiographical memories from only the most recent 2–5 years. To explain this pattern, memory theorists argue that the hippocampus acts as a temporary 'link' system for newly acquired memories: the individual elements constituting a new episode, such as images of people, places and fragments of conversation, are held to be stored in appropriate areas of sensory cortex but the hippocampal formation provides the essential link that binds the elements into a distinct episode. The hippocampus, it is argued, has limited neural space and most trivial memories fade so that space can be re-used. More significant events, which are rehearsed and refreshed by reminiscence, retelling or perhaps even dreaming, establish more permanent connections in the cortex and gradually become independent of the hippocampal formation, a process known as **consolidation.**

Recent findings in patients with apparently circumscribed damage to the hippocampus have cast doubt on this model. It appears that some hippocampal patients may have a temporally extensive retrograde memory loss encompassing the whole of their life. To explain this finding, opponents of the standard consolidation model argue that memory rehearsal and refreshment leads to the formation of multiple traces in the hippocampus itself (**the multiple trace model**) and that the extent of retrograde amnesia depends, therefore, upon the extent of hippocampal formation damage. Hence partial damage will cause a temporally limited retrograde loss whereas more severe damage will produce extensive remote memory loss. Upholders of the standard model argue that patients with temporally extensive loss must have damage to other brain structures. This controversy remains unresolved, although recent brain activation studies in normal subjects support the multiple trace position.

It also appears that structures closely related to the hippocampus, notably the entorhinal and perirhinal cortices, have a key role in aspects of memory previously ascribed to the hippocampus. The hippocampus itself is still thought to be critical for spatial memory and for so-called cross-modal association, for instance learning that a particular pattern or face occurred in a particular spatial location. By contrast, recognition memory depends more upon these parahippocampal structures.

Memory impairment is also a major and early feature of Alzheimer's disease and other dementing disorders. In Alzheimer's the situation is more complex than that in the amnestic syndrome. Each of the processes involved in long-term memory—encoding, consolidation, and retrieval—may be impaired. One of the hallmarks of early Alzheimer's is a very rapid forgetting of any new material; but there is also extensive retrograde amnesia, implying either problems with retrieval or a loss of stored information. Initially, short-term (working) memory may be normal but with disease progression this too becomes defective. In addition, semantic memory breaks down, so that the patients' database of knowledge about the world progressively declines, leading to a range of deficits, including diminished vocabulary, impaired word comprehension, and difficulty in naming objects.

Frontal lobe: attention, working memory and the temporal aspects of episodic memory

Patients with damage to the dorsolateral prefrontal cortex frequently complain of poor memory and forgetfulness, which is even more apparent to family members. Yet unlike patients with medial temporal lobe and diencephalic lesions they perform relatively well on standard memory tests: they are likely to show weak performance on word list learning tests and recall of stories but do much better on recognition-based memory tests. They cannot, therefore, be considered as classically amnesic. This discrepancy between symptoms and test performance can be understood in terms of the difference between the processes required for effective memory use and those involved in memory encoding, storage and consolidation. Another way of looking at this is to regard the prefrontal cortex as the conductor of the memory orchestra. Without a conductor there is chaos even although all of the players are present. In addition, the prefrontal cortex has a specific role in the temporal aspects of episodic memory. Patients with damage to this region mistake when they learnt various things, leading to a mix-up or conflation of past memories and a form of **confabulation**. Another more colourful form of confabulation, known as fantastic confabulation, is much rarer and occurs in the acute stages of Wernicke–Korsakoff syndrome and in patients with basal forebrain damage following subarachnoid haemorrhage and also after brain trauma. Such patients relate the occurrence of things that did not happen to them, for example, saying that they went to London last week and had tea with the Prime Minister.

Tests of anterograde episodic memory

Verbal

- Recall of complex verbal information such as stories (for example, the logical memory subtest of the Wechsler Memory Scales).
- Word-list learning (for example, the Rey Auditory Verbal Learning Test, and the California Verbal Learning Test).
- Recognition memory for newly encountered words (for example, Warrington's Recognition Memory Test).

Non-verbal

- Recall of geometric figures (for example, the Rey–Osterrieth Figure Test, and the Visual Reproduction and Figural Memory Subtests of the Wechsler Memory Scale).
- Recognition of newly encountered faces (for example, Warrington's Recognition Memory Test).
- Tests of spatial location recall [such as the Paired Associate Learning (PAL) test from CANTAB].

Memory batteries

- Weschler Memory Scales
- Rivermead Behavioural Memory Test
- The Doors and People Test

Tests of retrograde memory

Personal (autobiographical)

- The Autobiographical Memory interview, a structured interview which probes for the personal facts and episodes from three life-periods: school, early adult, and recent.

◆ Cued word association (Galton–Crovitz technique), which tests for personally experienced episodes evoked by a standard test of words (for example,
boat, train, baby, etc.), and is used in research projects on remote memory.

Semantic memory

The storage, maintenance, and retrieval of factual information and vocabulary
does not, in contrast to episodic memory, depend upon the limbic system. All
new facts and words are assumed to be learnt in the context of an episode; but
at some stage, perhaps with repeated rehearsal, they enter our fund of general
knowledge. Their retrieval then becomes independent of the personal and
time-tagged labels essential for recreating episodic memories. To illustrate this
difference consider attending a lecture on a new topic: recall of the information
is at first very dependent upon the context, and proceeds by reconstruction of
the events at the time of acquisition; with repeated exposure (or retrievals)
some of the information becomes part of our general store. Who can recall
where and when they first learnt the meaning of the word haemorrhage, or the
name of the capital of France? There is, however, recent evidence that children
with early life damage to their hippocampal system (developmental amnesia)
do acquire semantic knowledge even in the absence of a normally functioning
episodic memory system, suggesting that, with repeated exposure, non-
hippocampal parts of the temporal lobe can acquire new semantic memories.

It is important to point out that deficits of semantic memory do not simply
affect word-based knowledge (such as the ability to name objects or to produce
word definitions) but involve the fundamental knowledge-base underlying
word knowledge. Current cognitive psychology models hypothesize that there
is a central, amodal, integrative store which contains abstract representations.
These abstract representations are linked to modality-specific areas that contain lexical, sound, visual or tactile information (see Figure 1.8). Breakdown of
this central amodal store has differential effects on various modalities of
input. Patients invariably show greater deficits on word-based tasks because
the mapping from words to meaning is entirely arbitrary. Take for instance the
following words: echnida, platonic or ewer. There is no way of knowing which
of these words refers to an animal whereas sounds and pictures contain inherent
or deducible information.

The study of semantic memory is relatively recent, but current evidence
suggests that the anterior temporal neocortex, particularly in the left hemisphere, is the key integrative region linking other, more posterior, temporal
and parietal regions. Loss of semantic memory occurs as a result of extensive
destruction of this anterior temporal region, often from **herpes simplex** virus

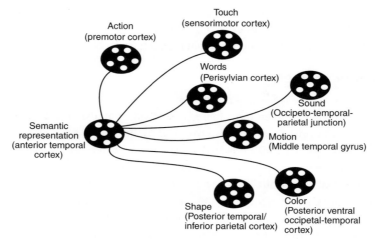

Fig. 1.8 Computational model of semantic memory. Reproduced with permission of Timothy Rogers and Karalyn Patterson.

encephalitis, or occasionally trauma or tumours. Progressive breakdown of semantic memory occurs in patients with Alzheimer's disease, who also have a severe impairment of episodic memory. The purest and most dramatic loss of semantic memory is seen in patients with semantic dementia (a variant of frontotemporal dementia) which is associated with circumscribed polar and inferior temporal lobe atrophy.

It seems that knowledge about different categories of things is stored separately, and in a highly organized fashion. A growing number of patients have been reported with so-called 'category-specific' semantic memory loss, affecting, for instance, knowledge about living, rather than man-made, things. Patients with even finer-grained deficits, involving for instance fruit and vegetables and not animals, have also been reported. A loss of knowledge about living or natural things is associated with temporal lobe damage (typical after **herpes simplex** encephalitis) whereas the rarer converse situation (impaired knowledge about man-made things) appears to be associated with damage to frontoparietal brain regions.

Another domain of increasing interest is the domain of person knowledge. This knowledge base enables us to name a picture of Tony Blair and to access information when given the name or hearing his voice, or to match the name and face. In contrast to general semantic knowledge, the right anterior temporal lobe appears to play a key role. Loss of person knowledge occurs in Alzheimer's disease, when it is associated with more general semantic memory breakdown, but can be seen as a relatively pure syndrome in patients with progressive right temporal lobe atrophy, which forms part of the spectrum of semantic dementia.

Disorders of semantic memory

1. Selective impairment (i.e. relative sparing of other cognitive abilities)
   - Semantic dementia (temporal lobe form of frontotemporal dementia)
   - **Herpes simplex** virus encephalitis (usually combined with amnesia)
   - Major head injury
   - Vascular lesions (for example, temporal lobe haemorrhage)
2. As part of more diffuse dementing disease
   - Alzheimer's disease
   - Vascular dementia

Tests of semantic memory

See Appendix for further details.

1. Tests of general knowledge and vocabulary (for example, the Information, Similarities, and Vocabulary subtests of the Wechsler Adult Intelligence Scale).
2. Category fluency (i.e. generation of exemplars from specified semantic categories such as animals, fruit, etc.).
3. Object naming to confrontation, which also depends upon intact perceptual and word retrieval abilities (for example, the Boston Naming Test, the Graded Naming Test).
4. Word-to-picture matching: picture-pointing in response to the spoken object name.
5. Tests of verbal knowledge (for example, 'What colour is a banana?'; 'Do canaries have wings?', etc.).
6. Non-verbal tests of semantic knowledge, such as those involving picture–picture matching (for example, the Pyramids and Palm Trees Test).
7. Person-based tasks, including naming photographs of famous people, providing information in response to names, matching faces and names, and picture–picture association tasks.

Semantic Memory Test Battery

In Cambridge we have developed a battery of tests based on the same 64 items (half living, half man-made) that includes the following subtests: category fluency, picture naming, word-to-picture matching, picture–picture association (The Camel and Cactus Test), picture and word sorting, repetition and generation of definitions from words (for a full description see p. 224).

Implicit memory

Both episodic and semantic memory are available to conscious access. We can reflect on both personally experienced events and our fund of knowledge of the world. However, other forms of learning occur to which we do not have conscious access. These have been termed 'implicit' or 'procedural' memory. Consider the act of learning to play a musical instrument, or learning to drive a car. Although we progressively acquire the motor skills involved in these tasks, we cannot fully explain the procedures, and improvement can only be tested practically. Another form of implicit learning goes under the term **priming**—in this, exposure to test stimuli improves subsequent performance, even if the subject has no conscious recollection of the initial exposure. For instance, on word-stem completion tests, subjects are first shown a list of words (for example, TRACE, BREEZE, METER, etc.), then asked to recall the list, and finally shown the initial three letters of each word (TRA, BRE, MET, etc.) and asked to complete each stem with the first word that comes to mind. Amnesic patients do well on the last task, although they have no memory of having seen the words. In a non-verbal priming test, fragmented-picture identification, subjects are shown a series of progressively less fragmented pictures of the same object, and asked to say as soon as they recognize the object. Normal subjects identify the objects much sooner (i.e. from more fragmented pictures) when re-shown the pictures. Amnesic patients demonstrate the same effect, although they deny having seen them before.

Implicit memory appears to depend neither upon the limbic system nor upon the temporal neocortex. Even patients with profound amnesia (for example, Korsakoff's syndrome) have spared implicit memory. Current evidence points to the basal ganglia as the key region for motor learning, although priming appears to depend upon cortical areas, and the cerebellum may also be important for some classical conditioned responses.

Implicit memory is not testable at the bedside. Questioning may reveal preservation of practical skills in patients with severe impairment of explicit memory; but the main reason for its inclusion here is to make readers aware of this important and rapidly expanding area of neuropsychological investigation.

Higher-Order Cognitive Function, Personality and Behaviour

The frontal lobes account for more than a third of the human neocortex (compared to 10% in non-human primates) and are undeniably crucial to the integrity of many aspects of 'higher-order' cognitive function, as well as to personality and behaviour. Damage to the prefrontal areas produces long-lasting and often devastating deficits. Yet it is notoriously difficult to define these cognitive domains accurately. Furthermore, there are no really satisfactory bedside methods of assessment. Even the neuropsychological tests traditionally described as so-called 'frontal lobe tasks' are crude, and do not capture many of the behavioural aspects of frontal dysfunction. Here, history taking from informants and clinical observation are especially important.

Cognitive functions attributed to the frontal lobes

Adaptive behaviour:

- Abstract conceptual ability
- Set-shifting/mental flexibility
- Inhibitory control
- Problem solving and strategy formation
- Planning
- Self-monitoring
- Initiation
- Sequencing of behaviour
- Decision making
- Temporal-order judgements
- Personality, especially drive, motivation, and inhibition
- Social behaviour including theory of mind
- Affect
- Motivation

For clinical purposes these diverse abilities can be considered under two main headings which correspond to anatomical subdivisions of the prefrontal cortex:

1. Executive abilities related to the dorsolateral prefrontal cortex.
2. Social cognition, inhibitory control and emotion related to orbitomesial regions.

Executive abilities

To be effective, behaviour must be appropriate, modifiable, motivated, and free from interference and disruptive impulsive responses. If responses are to be appropriately adapted, changes in the environment need to be monitored and, if possible, anticipated. Patients with frontal lobe damage fail to anticipate changes, show poor planning ability, and do not learn from their errors. Planning is a particularly important practical function, since many complex behaviours—such as organizing a household, or holding down a job of work—require the planning and sequencing of behaviours, as well as the setting of goals. Frontal patients are especially poor at self-guided learning and goal setting. They perform normally on externally driven tasks, but are very poor at self-motivated learning. There is a striking vulnerability to interference from irrelevant stimuli, resulting in distractibility and the intrusion of unwanted responses. They also show a tendency to perseverate. Perseveration can be observed on motor tasks (such as learning a sequence of hand movements, as in the Luria three-step test described on p. 125), when a compulsive repetition of movement is observed. Perseverative tendencies can also be seen on cognitive tests independent of motor activity, where subjects perseverate correct and incorrect responses. There is also an inability to shift from one task to another, and a peculiar mental stickiness described as 'stimulus-bound' behaviour. Many of the above cognitive functions are necessary for effective problem solving and it is, therefore, not surprising that frontal lobe damage results in severe deficits in solving problems, deducing concepts, and making analogies.

A classic test of strategy formation and shifting is the Wisconsin Card Sorting Test (WCST) which requires elements of hypothesis testing, shifting and flexibility. The WCST forms the basis of a more sophisticated set-shifting task in the computerized CANTAB battery. Complex frontal executive abilities are also assessed by tests of fluid (as opposed to crystallized) intelligence such as Raven's Progressive Matrices or Catell's test of G. Another popular test of problem solving is the Tower of London (originally Hanoi) task which is also available in a modified form as part of the CANTAB battery.

The inability to initiate and monitor cognitive strategies can also be tested by verbal fluency tasks. In the supermarket fluency test, patients are asked to list items which can be bought in a supermarket. In category fluency tests they are asked to list as many exemplars as possible from a given category (for example, animals, fruit, vegetables, etc.) in a limited time-period, usually 1 min. Letter fluency tests require subjects to generate as many words as possible beginning with certain letters (for instance, F, A and S). Frontal patients show severe impoverishment in the generation of exemplars, impaired search strategies, and a tendency to repeat the same item (see p. 122 for details of tests).

Although not involved in the laying down and storage of long-term memory traces, the frontal lobes are important for certain aspects of memory retrieval, particularly when temporal-order judgements are required (see p. 17).

One of the components of working memory, the central executor, also depends critically upon the frontal lobes (see p. 8). Patients with frontal lobe dysfunction may, therefore, be impaired on simple tests of short-term (working) memory (for example, reverse digit span); but they also show very marked deficits on dual-task performance tests that place heavy demands upon working memory, such as simultaneous digit span and manual tracking.

Social cognition, inhibitory control and emotion

Patients with damage to the orbitomesial frontal lobe suffer profound changes in personality and behaviour yet may perform normally on all the tests of executive function discussed above. This dissociation is exemplified by the famous case of Phineas Gage who suffered major alterations in social cognition after a tamping iron penetrated his orbital frontal lobe and exited the top of his skull. Having previously been a responsible and well-adjusted, hardworking, conscientious worker he became feckless, irresponsible, indecisive, emotionally cold and impulsive. Such cases are still seen today following road traffic accidents or surgery for orbital meningiomas but in neurological practice this constellation is most often seen in association with progressive frontal lobe degeneration as part of frontotemporal dementia (also known as Pick's disease).

Considerable progress has been made over the past two decades in our understanding of these changes. The orbital cortex has reciprocal connections with the amygdala, temporal pole and insula cortex. Together these structures constitute a critical circuit involved in emotion judgement and responsiveness. One important hypothesis, advocated by Antonio Demasio and colleagues, is that the orbital cortex contains so-called **somatic markers**, which are evoked by a range of sensory experiences and give rise to inner feelings necessary for normal mature human interactions. Patients with damage to components of this circuit may be impaired in their perception of emotions from facial expressions or from voice, whereas others can perceive emotions but have lost the appropriate valence associated with these perceptions leading to a form of acquired psychopathy.

Another theoretical advance has been the development of the concept of **theory of mind**, sometimes also referred to as mentalizing ability. This concept grew out of observations in individuals with autism and Asperger's syndrome who are unable to appreciate the mental state of others. Functional brain-imaging studies localize theory-of-mind abilities to the orbital and medial frontal cortices plus the superior temporal sulcus. A loss of empathy and humour appreciation is thought to reflect defective theory of mind and is common in patients with frontal pathology. Another striking similarity between individuals with autism and patients with orbitomesial frontal damage is the occurrence of stereotypical ritualized behaviours akin to obsessive-compulsive disorder. Patients with frontotemporal dementia indulge in repetitive, complex patterns of ritualized behaviours such as hoarding and collecting.

These behaviours are also seen in some patients with Parkinson's disease who abuse dopaminergic therapies and are referred to in this context as punding behaviours.

Alterations in food preference, mainly towards sweet foods, and satiety are also common features of frontotemporal dementia and again reflect disruption of circuits involving the orbital frontal cortex, the amygdala and the gustatory cortex in the insula.

Another hallmark of orbitofrontal damage is loss of inhibitory control. This results in a tendency to react immediately, and usually inappropriately, to external stimuli. Irascibility and verbal aggression are common.

A final aspect of cognition frequently impaired after mesial frontal lobe damage is motivation. Apathy is a very common feature and its most extreme form results in an abulic state of motionless mutism. This is rare but occurs after anterior cerebral artery occlusion or neurosurgical interventions. Less profound states of apathy are very common in Alzheimer's disease, frontotemporal dementia and the parkinsonian syndromes especially progressive supranuclear palsy.

Frontal lobes: applied anatomy

The frontal lobes proper can be subdivided into five major areas (see Figure 1.9):

1. The motor area (primary motor cortex), which occupies the precentral gyrus.

2. The supplementary motor area, which lies immediately anterior to the motor strip, and serves to co-ordinate and plan motor activity.

3. The frontal eye fields, which mediate volitional and involuntary eye movements in the contralateral direction, and are also important for spatial attention.

4. Broca's area, which occupies the inferior prefrontal region in the dominant, usually left, hemisphere.

5. The prefrontal cortex proper which in turn has three subdivisions: dorsolateral, orbital and mesial each with distinct functions as discussed above.

In keeping with its role as the chief executive officer of intellectual function, the prefrontal cortex is richly connected to virtually all other subordinate cortical and subcortical structures. It receives inputs from all unimodal association areas (visual, auditory, haptic, olfactory) and the other multimodal association areas (i.e. the posterior parietal and ventral temporal lobes), as well as from the limbic structures. Major afferent projections arise from the

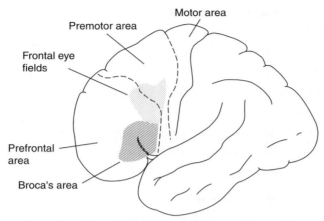

Fig. 1.9 Dorsolateral frontal cortex with functional areas.

dorsomedial nucleus of the thalamus and basal ganglia. This accounts for the 'frontal lobe' or dysexecutive deficits that typically occur in the subcortical dementia syndrome associated with basal ganglia disorders (for example, Huntington's disease, progressive supranuclear palsy, and Parkinson's disease), and in lesions of the thalamus.

The orbitomesial frontal cortex is richly interconnected with the polar parts of the temporal lobe and the amygdala as discussed above.

Disorders of frontal lobe function

Degenerative

- Frontotemporal dementia (Pick's disease)
- Alzheimer's disease later in the course of the disease

Vascular

- Bilateral anterior cerebral artery infarction
- Following subarachnoid haemorrhage (anterior communicating artery aneurysms)

Structural

- Major closed head injury (orbital, frontal and temporal lobes most frequently damaged)
- Tumours (butterfly glioma and subfrontal meningioma)
- Surgical resection
- Frontal leucotomy

Deafferentation from basal ganglia disorders

Examples include:

- Huntington's disease
- Parkinson's disease
- Progressive supranuclear palsy (Steele–Richardson–Olszewski syndrome)
- Wilson's disease
- Vascular: in multi-infarct and diffuse subcortical leucoaryosis dementia frontal features are a major component
- Multiple Sclerosis and the leucodystrophies

Tests of frontal lobe function

See Chapter 4 and Appendix for further details.

- Verbal fluency (category and letter-based tests)
- Analogies and sequencing (for example, the Similarities and Picture Arrangement subtests from the WAIS, and Raven's Matrices)
- Problem-solving [for example, the Tower of London (or Hanoi) test, which requires subjects to move coloured discs onto three posts to obtain target designs in a set number of moves]
- Proverb interpretation
- Cognitive Estimates Test
- Trail Making Test
- Set-shifting (for example, the Wisconsin Card Sorting Test and the ID-ED test of the CANTAB)
- Motor sequencing (for example, alternating hand movements and the Luria three-step test)
- Decision making tests such as the Iowa Gambling test

Chapter 2

Delirium and Dementia

Having considered the three major areas of cognition with a distributed neural basis—attention, memory, and executive function—it is now appropriate to describe briefly delirium and dementia, which almost invariably affect one or more of these cognitive domains. Patients with one, or both, of these conditions constitute the commonest presentation in behavioural neurology and in geriatric psychiatry.

Delirium

Delirium may be defined as a transient organic mental syndrome of acute onset, characterized by marked attentional abnormalities, an impairment in global cognitive functions, perceptual disturbances, increased and/or decreased psychomotor activity, a disordered sleep–wake cycle, and a tendency to marked fluctuations (see Table 2.1).

Several components of this definition deserve further comment. Although delirium is a syndrome with certain core characteristics, the clinical manifestations may vary widely. The features vary between patients and often in a single patient over the course of 24 h. The onset is always acute or subacute, occurring over hours or days and often at night. The total duration rarely exceeds weeks. The prognosis clearly depends upon the aetiology but if the underlying cause is cured then a complete recovery can be expected. The aspects of cognition principally involved are those with a distributed cerebral basis—attention, memory, and higher-order executive functions (for example, planning, problem solving, abstraction, sequencing, etc.). Deficits of the more localized cognitive functions, such as language and praxis, may also be seen; but the distributed-function deficits always dominate. Clouding of consciousness is no longer included in contemporary definitions of delirium, for the reasons discussed below.

Attention and memory

A disturbance in attention is the most striking and consistent abnormality: patients are unable to generate and sustain attention to external stimuli, and have problems with shifting attention appropriately. They appear distractible, and easily lose the thread of conversations. Accordingly, there is severe impairment

Table 2.1 Features of delirium (acute confusional state)

1. Reduced ability to maintain attention to external stimuli, and to shift attention to new stimuli appropriately

2. Disorganized thinking, as indicated by rambling, irrelevant, or incoherent speech

3. Memory impairment: poor registration and retention of new material

4. Perceptual distortions, leading to misidentification, illusions, and hallucinations

5. Increased or decreased psychomotor activity

6. A disturbed sleep–wake cycle

7. Disorientation in time, and often in place

8. Changes in mood, such as anxiety, depression, or lability

9. A tendency to fluctuations and nocturnal exacerbation

on tests requiring sustained concentration and the manipulation of material, such as serial subtraction of 7s, recitation of the months of the year or days of the week in reverse order, and digit span. Another good test for sustained attention is the ability to generate words beginning with certain letters (for example, F, A and S) or from specific semantic categories (for example, animals, fruit, etc.). Patients with impaired attention produce few exemplars, tend to perseverate, and revert to a previous category.

Disorientation in time is almost always present at some time during the illness. Disturbed appreciation of the passage of time is universal. Disorientation for place, and still later for person, may follow with worsening of perceptual and cognitive organization.

The disturbance in memory is largely secondary to diminished attention. Incoming sensory material is poorly attended to and registered. Immediate repetition of a name and address is characteristically defective, and patients need multiple presentations before simple material is repeated correctly. Confabulatory responses may be seen. Retrograde memory is reasonably intact if the patient's attention can be focused and sustained. On recovery from delirium there is typically a dense amnesic gap for the period of the illness, although where fluctuation has been marked islands of memory may remain.

Thinking

The organization and content of thought processes are invariably affected in delirium. Even in mild cases there is difficulty in formulating complex ideas and sustaining a logical train of thought. Attempts at history taking reveal the muddled, illogical and disjointed nature of the patient's thinking. The capacity to select thoughts and maintain their organization and sequence for the purpose of problem solving and planning is drastically reduced. Concept formation is impaired, with a tendency to concrete thinking. These deficits are apparent on bedside testing of proverb interpretation, similarity judgement, generation of word definitions, and category fluency.

The content of thought may be dominated by the patient's concerns, wishes, and fantasies. There is often a dream-like quality to the patient's thinking. Delusions (i.e. false beliefs incongruent with the patient's cultural and educational background) are often present. These are usually fleeting, poorly elaborated, and inconsistent. A paranoid persecutory content is most common. For instance, patients may believe that they are about to be killed by the nurse or doctors, or that close family members have been murdered. Delusions, illusions and hallucinations frequently occur together.

Disorders of perception

Perception in this context refers to the ability to extract information from the environment and one's own body and to integrate it in a meaningful way. Attentional processes play a crucial role in the perception of sensory information, and the ubiquitous attentional disorder seen in delirium probably underlies many of the perceptual disturbances seen. Vision and hearing are most commonly affected. Disturbance of vision may lead to micropsia, macropsia, or distortions of shape and position, fragmentation, apparent movement, or autoscopy (the perception of seeing oneself from outside the body). Sounds may be accentuated or distorted. Body image may be affected, causing a perceived alteration of size, shape, or position. Bizarre reduplicative phenomena may be reported—for example, when the patient believes that there are two identical hospital wards and they are being moved from one to the other. Feelings of depersonalization and unreality are very common.

Illusions—the misperception of external stimuli—are frequent, and most often involve the visual modality. Patients may mistake spots on the wall for insects, or patterns on the bed-cover for snakes. Illusions may be interwoven with delusions, so that ward sounds are incorporated into persecutory plots. Family members and staff may be misidentified.

Hallucinations are also common. Visual hallucinations are most characteristic, and range in complexity from simple shapes and patterns to fully formed objects, animals, mythological or ghostlike apparitions, and panoramic scenes. They are often brightly coloured, with elements that change in position, size, and number. The hallucinated material may be grossly distorted, as for example in Lilliputian hallucinations, where minute people or objects appear. Combined auditory and visual hallucinations are also frequent. Tactile hallucinations take the form of crawling, creeping, or burning sensations.

Delusions of infestation or sexual interference may accompany such sensations. Olfactory hallucinations are also described. In general, hallucinations occur in patients with the hyperalert (see below) variant of delirium. Withdrawal from alcohol and sedative-hypnotics seems particularly prone to produce frank hallucinations.

The sleep–wake cycle

A disruption of the normal circadian sleep–wake cycle is a consistent feature of delirium, and is considered by some authors to be central to the pathogenesis of the syndrome. Insomnia, with a worsening of confusion at night, is common. Other features include daytime sleepiness, dreamlike states with vivid imagery, and a breakdown in the ability to distinguish between dreams and reality.

Electroencephalogram (EEG) tracings taken during the day show fluctuations, and transition from wakefulness, light, rapid eye movement (REM), and deep sleep. Night-time recordings show a loss of the normal orderly progression of the stages of sleep. Maintenance of the normal sleep–wake cycle depends upon the complex interaction of neurotransmitter systems that constitute the reticular activating system (see p. 3).

Psychomotor behaviour, emotion, and mood

A disturbance of general psychomotor activity is virtually always present in delirium. Two contrasting patterns may be distinguished; but not infrequently patients alternate between the two.

In the **hyperalert** variant, the patient is restless, excitable, and vigilant. He or she responds promptly, and often excessively, to any stimulus. Speech is voluble and pressured. Shouting, laughing, and crying are common. There is increased physical activity often with repetitive purposeless behaviour, such as groping or picking. Often the patient tries to get out of bed, and attempts at restraint may produce violent outbursts. Autonomic signs of hyperarousal, such as tachycardia, sweating and pupillary dilatation can be observed. Vivid hallucinations tend to be seen most often in patients with this variant.

Patients with the **hypoalert** variant are, by contrast, quiet and motionless; they drift off to sleep if stimulated, and display reduced psychomotor activity. Speech is typically sparse and slow; answers to questions are stereotypic, and often incoherent. Despite outward appearances the patient may be experiencing delusions and hallucinations, although they are less frequent than in the hyperalert variant.

Emotional disturbances are very frequent, and may vary from euphoria to depression. A state of perplexity, with apathy and indifference, is perhaps most often seen. Lability is common, and the patient may suddenly become fearful, angry and aggressive.

Clouding of consciousness

This term was traditionally included in descriptions of delirium, but has been dropped from current definitions. There is no generally accepted definition of consciousness; and 'clouding' is an even vaguer term. Consciousness may be considered in a narrow sense to mean a level of wakefulness and response to gross external stimuli. Although patients with delirium may be drowsy and show reduced response when stimulated, often they are fully awake, and may even be hyperalert. In a broader sense, consciousness has been used to describe the capacity to engage in complex and appropriate thought, to fix, sustain, and shift attention, and to judge the passage of time. Impairment or clouding of consciousness, used in this sense, is thus no more than a metaphor referring to the set of cognitive and attentional deficits that constitute the core of the syndrome of delirium.

Causes of delirium

A variety of factors can cause delirium (see Table 2.2).

Table 2.2 Causes of delirium (acute confusional states)

1. Metabolic encephalopathies
   - Acid–base or electrolyte imbalance
   - Hypoglycaemia
   - Hypoxia, hypercapnia
   - Hepatic or renal failure
   - Wernicke's encephalopathy and other B-vitamin deficiencies
   - Endocrine disorders, for example Cushing's disease, Addison's disease
   - Porphyria

2. Intoxication by drugs and poisons
   - A wide range of drugs, including anticholinergics, hypnotic-sedatives, anti-parkinsonian agents, anticonvulsants, digoxin, etc.
   - Alcohol, illicit drugs, and inhalants
   - Industrial poisons

3. Withdrawal syndromes, especially from alcohol and hypnotic-sedatives

4. Infections, both intracranial (meningitis, encephalitis) and systemic

5. Multifocal and diffuse brain disease
   - Anoxia, fat embolism
   - Vasculitis
   - Cerebrovascular disease
   - Raised intracranial pressure, hydrocephalus

6. Head trauma

7. Epilepsy, including post-ictal states and non-convulsive status

8. Focal brain lesions, particularly to the brain stem or right hemisphere

Cortical versus subcortical dementia

A recently proposed division of primary degenerative diseases, which has proved theoretically and practically useful, is between those which affect primarily the cerebral cortex and those in which the major pathological impact is on subcortical structures. The reason for the cognitive impairment in the former is obvious. In the subcortical dementias, the major impact is thought to result from a loss of the normal regulatory effect of subcortical structures on the cortex, particularly the prefrontal area. The term subcortical dementia was initially applied to the cognitive syndrome seen in progressive supranuclear palsy and Huntington's disease, but has been subsequently applied to a range of basal ganglia and white matter diseases (see Table 2.4).

Alzheimer's disease is the prototypical example of a cortical dementia in which disturbances of memory, language and visuo-spatial abilities predominate (see Table 2.5). Attention and frontal executive functions are relatively well preserved in the early stages. The slowing of cognitive processes (bradyphrenia), change in personality, and mood disturbances which characterize subcortical dementias are less prominent until late in the disease. Marked impairment in episodic memory is practically always the earliest feature in Alzheimer's disease. The amnesia reflects a failure of encoding and a very rapid forgetting of any new material. Recall and recognition are both severely affected. Remote memory is also affected, with a temporal gradient, in that early-life memories are relatively spared. Within the domain of language, aphasia occurs fairly early in the course: reflecting a breakdown in the semantic components of language, with relative sparing of phonology and syntax; word-finding difficulty in spontaneous conversation, impaired naming on formal tests and impaired generation of exemplars on category fluency testing (for example, on animals, or fruit) are consistent early findings; the picture in more advanced Alzheimer's disease has been likened to transcortical sensory aphasia (see p. 68).

Table 2.4 Cortical and subcortical dementias

Cortical dementias	Subcortical dementias
Alzheimer's disease	Progressive supranuclear palsy (Steele–Richardson–Olszewski syndrome)
Creutzfeldt–Jakob disease	Huntington's disease
Parkinson's disease	Wilson's disease
Frontotemporal dementia	Normal pressure hydrocepalus
	White matter diseases (leucodystrophies and multiple sclerosis)
	AIDS encephalopathy

Table 2.5 Summary of features of cortical and subcortical dementias

Function	Cortical dementia (e.g. Alzheimer's disease)	Subcortical dementia (e.g. Huntinton's disease)
Alertness	Normal	Marked 'slowing up' (bradyphrenia)
Attention	Intact in early stages	Impaired
Episodic memory	Severe amnesia	Forgetfulness due to poor encoding; recognition better than recall
Frontal 'executive'	Normal until late function	Typically impaired from onset
Personality	Preserved	Apathetic, inert
Language	Aphasic features	Normal, except for reduced output and dysarthria
Praxis	Impaired	Normal
Visuo-spatial and perceptual abilities	Impaired	Impaired

In subcortical dementia, as exemplified by Huntington's disease or progressive supranuclear palsy, impairment in attentional control and frontal 'executive' functions predominates (see Table 2.5). Patients appear characteristically 'slowed up' (bradyphrenic), with a marked deficit in the retrieval of information. Spontaneous speech is reduced, and answers to questions are slow and laconic. Changes in mood, personality, and social conduct are very common. Patients are often inert, indifferent, and uninterested. Memory is impaired, mainly as a result of reduced attention leading to poor encoding of new material; but the severe amnesia which typifies Alzheimer's disease is not seen in the early stages. Recognition is typically much better than spontaneous recall. It is easy to overestimate the degree of cognitive impairment in patients with subcortical dementia, and performance usually improves with persistence and encouragement. Features of focal cortical dysfunction, such as aphasia, apraxia and agnosia, are characteristically absent, at least in the earlier stages. But visuo-spatial and perceptual abnormalities can be demonstrated fairly consistently.

It should be pointed out that not all dementias can be fitted neatly into this dichotomy. In vascular dementia, for example, subcortical features predominate, owing to multiple lacunar lesions in the basal ganglia or diffuse white matter pathology; but there is often evidence of focal cortical damage.

Another recently identified disease in which a mixture of cortical and subcortical features occurs is dementia with Lewy bodies (DLB). The pathological hallmark of Parkinson's disease is the presence of Lewy bodies in the substantia nigra. In DLB these inclusion bodies are found throughout the cortex. Patients display a variety of symptoms with characteristic subcortical deficits (particularly poor executive ability and attention), and features of cortical dysfunction, the latter implicating parieto-occipital regions.

Frontotemporal dementia also presents a problem as patients with the behavioural form present with changes in personality and social conduct and classic cortical features.

Alzheimer's disease

In 1906 Alois Alzheimer reported the case of a woman aged 51 years, Auguste D, with severe amnesia, aphasia and hallucinations who, at post-mortem, showed silver-staining plaques and tangles. For the next 50 years it was considered to be a rare cause of presenile dementia but it gradually became clear that identical pathology was responsible for the majority of cases of late-onset dementia as well. The prevalence rises considerably with advancing age, doubling every 5 years. The distinction between presenile and senile dementia is, in general, no longer valid except that a proportion of young-onset patients have genetic mutations: most commonly involving the Presenilin I (PSI) gene but occasionally the Amyloid Precursor Protein (APP) gene. Some PSI mutations are associated with spastic paraparesis. Controversy exists on whether there are other clinical hallmarks of familial Alzheimer's disease (AD). It is generally held that young-onset cases have a more rapid progression. It should be noted, in passing, that even in early-onset cases only a minority are found to have a gene mutation although the proportion increases considerably in patients with a strong family history of early-onset dementia.

The defining characteristic of AD remains the neuropathology, which consists of intraneuronal tangles of paired helical filaments (PHFs) and extraneuronal plaques containing an amyloid core. PHFs are regarded as more important for the genesis of symptoms and arise initially in the parahippocampal region (specifically the entorhinal cortex) before spreading to the hippocampus proper and the posterior association cortices. The staging of pathological changes proposed by Braak and Braak (see Figure 2.1) has formed the basis of our understanding of the evolution of the cognitive deficits seen in AD.

Since there is no definitive way of establishing the diagnosis in life, it has become common practice to apply the term 'dementia of Alzheimer type' (DAT). However, with the use of strict research criteria (such as the NINCDS-ADRDA)

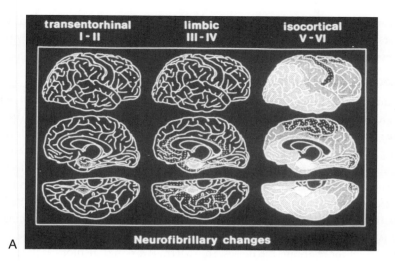

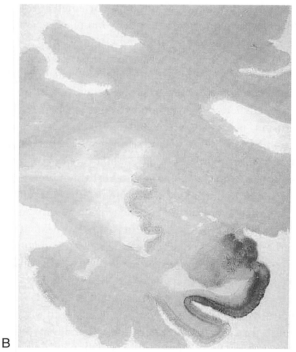

Fig. 2.1 (a) Braak and Braak Stages: cartoon of tangle spread. (b) Brain slice: thin slice of brain through the temporal lobes showing staining with silver, indicating the density of Alzheimer pathology in the medial temporal lobe.

an accurate diagnosis can be made in at least 80% of cases. Alzheimer's disease does not begin with a 'global' loss of intellectual function, but generally progresses in a predictable fashion through the following stages.

Stage 1: Mild cognitive impairment

From the onset there is almost invariably episodic memory impairment, with features similar to those resulting from other causes of the amnesic syndrome (see p. 15). Anterograde amnesia results from poor encoding and rapid forgetting of new material. Retrieval may also be poor with some improvement on cueing or on recognition-based tests. The amnesia is typically global, affecting verbal and non-verbal (faces and shapes etc.) material, but patients with more selective deficits are seen. Tests of associative learning, such as the Paired Associate Learning (PAL) test from the CANTAB battery, appear particularly sensitive. The retrograde memory loss has a temporally graded pattern, with sparing of more distant memories. Short-term (working) memory as judged by digit span is generally normal. Patients are often well oriented at this stage. Language is typically normal on informal assessment, but poor generation of exemplars on category fluency (for example in naming animals, fruit, etc.) may be found: a dissociation between category fluency (impaired) and letter fluency (preserved) is highly suggestive of AD or semantic dementia. Visuo-spatial functioning is good. Patients perform normally on simple executive tests but more complex tasks may reveal deficits. Slowing on timed tasks (such as Trails B or digit-symbol substitution) is present in a proportion of cases from an early stage. Social rapport and personality are well preserved, thus often masking the severity of the amnestic problem. Apathy and irritability are the commonest neurobehavioural symptoms and can be found in a fairly high proportion of cases. Many patients suffer from low mood which can be interpreted either in terms of a psychological reaction or a disturbance of neurochemical systems.

Patients typically score above the accepted cut-off on the Mini-Mental State Examination (MMSE) and continue to perform basic activities of daily living normally. They cannot, therefore, be regarded as 'demented' in the classic sense. A number of different labels have been applied to patients in this amnestic prodrome of dementia proper, the most popular of which is **mild cognitive impairment** (MCI). The prognosis for patients with MCI varies depending on the criteria used in different studies, but a generally agreed figure for conversion to frank dementia is in the order of 10–20% per annum. Whether all such patients eventually convert remains a contentious issue but certainly the majority will do so within 5 years of follow-up. We have followed patients for 8 years before conversion to dementia. Current research criteria for MCI are as shown in Table 2.6.

Table 2.6 Criteria for mild cognitive impairment

1. Complaints of poor memory corroborated by an informant
2. Objective evidence of episodic memory impairment, generally >1.5 standard deviations below controls' mean level on a standard test such as story recall or word list learning
3. Largely intact general (non-memory) cognitive abilities
4. Normal activities of daily living
5. Not reaching DSM IV criteria for dementia

Stage 2: Mild-to-moderate dementia

Worsening memory abilities and impaired attention result in marked temporal disorientation and patients retain very little new information. Remote memory is impaired and deficits in short-term (working) memory are found. Distractibility, poor attention and problems with frontal executive function are ubiquitous. Breakdown of semantic memory results in diminished vocabulary, word-finding difficulty, and semantic paraphasic errors in spontaneous conversation, very poor naming ability, reduced generation of exemplars on category fluency testing, and a loss of general knowledge. Difficulties with comprehension of syntactically complex sentences and in performing phonological tasks also occur. Visuo-spatial deficits are readily apparent. Relatives report a general slowing or ageing with difficulty performing everyday activities. Neuropsychiatric symptoms are increasingly prominent with apathy, mood disturbance, irritability and agitation, delusions and sometimes hallucinations. Social rapport is still partly preserved, thus patients appear (superficially) to be reasonably intact; but beneath the social veneer they are empty shells.

Stage 3: Advanced dementia

Marked global loss in all areas of intellectual function—amnesia, aphasia, agnosia, etc. There is also progressive disintegration of personality. Incontinence, disorders of social conduct and aggressive behaviour are common. Increasing dependence leads to death.

Atypical Alzheimer's disease

Although the majority of patients present with episodic memory loss as their most prominent deficit, it is clear that there are two major variants: progressive aphasia and progressive visuo-spatial impairment. In patients with the former, language variant may resemble those with semantic dementia or with progressive non-fluent aphasia but the language syndrome is hardly ever as pure and other subtle deficits in visual memory and visuo-spatial deficits are usually present. Note that in aphasic patients it is very difficult to assess episodic memory, so reliance must be placed upon non-verbal tasks such as recall of abstract shapes, recognition of faces and spatial learning.

Patients with the visual variant of Alzheimer's disease present with difficulty navigating in unfamiliar environments, problems reaching and grasping objects, various complex visual symptoms including neglect and, on examination, features of Balint's syndrome are present (see p. 91). Magnetic resonance imaging (MRI) scans in such patients reveal occipitoparietal atrophy which has led to the adoption of the label **posterior cortical atrophy**. Memory, language and insight are often very well preserved. As this disorder progresses patients may become functionally blind. Apraxia is also common. The differentiation of posterior cortical atrophy from corticobasal degeneration (CBD) and dementia with Lewy bodies can be very difficult.

Neuroimaging in Alzheimer's disease

The most important role of imaging in patients with suspected Alzheimer's disease is to exclude other potentially treatable disorders (see below). Computed tomography (CT) scanning is generally unremarkable in the early stages. Even standard clinical MRI scans may be passed as normal. Research MRI with coronal cuts will show hippocampal atrophy from an early stage although these changes are subtle and hard to detect unless volumetric analyses are used. Functional scans [single photon emission computed tomography (SPECT) or positron emission tomography (PET)] reveal more striking changes with posterior cingulate and/or bilateral parieto-temporal hypometabolism.

Frontotemporal dementia (Pick's disease)

Arnold Pick, a contemporary of Alois Alzheimer, recognized in the early years of the 20th century the existence of patients with both progressive fluent aphasia and personality deterioration associated with focal atrophy confined, at least initially, to either the frontal or temporal lobes. This is now referred to as frontotemporal dementia (FTD), or sometimes frontotemporal lobar degeneration (FTLD). Characteristic pathological changes, distinct from that seen in Alzheimer's disease—silver positive (argyrophilic) inclusions known as Pick bodies—were subsequently identified, although it was later found that these histological changes are present in a minority of cases.

The past decade has seen an explosion of knowledge concerning the pathology and genetics of FTD. Three major pathological subforms are now recognized.

1. Tau-positive cases. This category includes cases with classic Pick's disease who have tau-positive intraneuronal Pick bodies and ballooned achromatic

neurons (Pick cells). Also included under this heading are patients with tau-positive pathology who lack Pick bodies but show diffuse tau-positive staining; the majority of inherited cases with mutations of the tau gene on chromosome 17 fall in this category, as do patients with corticobasal degeneration (CBD) who have ballooned achromatic neurons and tau-positive astrocytic tangles and patients with argyrophilic grain disease which is characterized by diffuse, small, punctate, tau-positive inclusions in the hippocampus and hypothalamus.

2. Ubiquitin-positive tau-negative cases. These inclusions were first identified in the context of motor neuron disease (MND) and then subsequently in patients with FTD in association with MND. More recently, FTD patients without MND have been found to have the same inclusions, typically in the dentate gyrus. Recent studies suggest that this variant is as common as the tau-positive form.

3. Finally there are rare tau-negative and ubiquitin-negative cases. These patients have the same distribution of atrophy and cell loss but lack any distinctive inclusions on immunohistology.

A high proportion of younger-onset dementia cases, seen in specialist clinics, have FTD. Two recent UK-based epidemiological studies have shown that, under the age of 65 years, FTD is almost as common as Alzheimer's disease. Up to a third of patients have a positive family history using the broad inclusion criteria of a relative with dementia, Parkinson's disease or motor neuron disease. Patients from an established kindred with more than one first-degree relative affected are rarer. A proportion of these patients (with tau-positive inclusions pathology) are found to have a mutation of the tau gene on chromosome 17, and very recently a second significant gene mutation has been found in families with ubiquitin-positive inclusion involving the progranulin gene also on chromosome 17.

There is growing awareness of the overlap between FTD and both MND and CBD: around 10% of patients with FTD develop clinically overt MND, usually of the bulbar type. These patients typically have rapidly progressive FTD with prominent behavioural changes as well as aphasia and sometimes psychotic phenomena. Within 12 months they develop features of MND. Conversely, a small, and yet to be fully defined, proportion of patients with MND also develops FTD.

Although CBD was initially characterized by asymmetric parkinsonism with severe limb apraxia, alien limb phenomena, falls and myoclonus, it is now clear that many (if not all) cases with CBD develop cognitive deficits, usually characterized by a progressive non-fluent aphasia with marked word finding

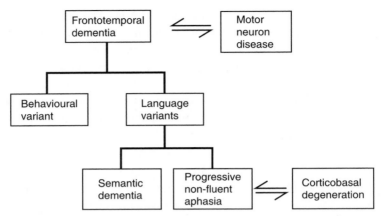

Fig. 2.2 Relationship between frontotemporal dementia, motor neuron disease and corticobasal degeneration.

and phonological deficits together with frontal executive problems reflecting involvement of the parietal and dorsolateral prefrontal cortices. Visuo-spatial impairment is also common in CBD unlike the other FTD syndromes.

The relationship between FTD syndromes, MND and CBD is illustrated in Figure 2.2.

Behavioural (frontal) presentation

This is the commonest variant of FTD and presents with changes in personality and social conduct (see Table 2.7). Patients become unconcerned, lacking in initiative, motivation, judgement and forethought and neglect their personal responsibilities, leading to mismanagement of domestic and financial affairs. Medical referral may occur following demotion, dismissal from work

Table 2.7 Key behavioural characteristics of frontotemporal dementia

1. Loss of social awareness and insight
2. Disinhibition and impulsivity
3. Apathy, inertia and aspontaneity
4. Mental rigidity and inflexibility
5. Personal neglect and declining self-care
6. Stereotypic behaviours and rituals
7. Change in eating habits and food preference
8. Loss of empathy and mentalizing ability

or increasing marital disharmony. Patients are typically unaware of these changes. A common early symptom is a lack of understanding of social conventions with reduced courtesy. Social *faux pas* become gradually more glaring. An indifference to the feelings of others with impaired empathy is very common.

Patients typically neglect personal hygiene and need to be encouraged to change their clothes and to wash. Changes in eating and drinking are very common. Over-eating and especially a craving for sweet foods may lead relatives to ration food. Food fads are common involving sweet, and highly flavoured, foods. Excessive and indiscriminate eating leads to obesity. Altered sexual behaviour is common which may take the form of loss of libido. Conversely some patients may make inappropriate sexual advances. Patients may be over-active, restless, distractible and disinhibited. Alternatively they may show apathy, inertia and aspontaneity. Often patients alternate from one to the other, dependent on the environmental situation.

Increasing inflexibility and adoption of fixed daily routines is very common. Activities often acquire a marked stereotypic quality. Patients may clock-watch, carrying out a particular activity at precisely the same time every day. Wandering may involve completion of an identical route at exactly the same time every day. Some patients constantly repeat the same phrase or sentence.

Establishing a definitive diagnosis can be very difficult as patients can appear normal and perform well on standard screening cognitive instruments such as the MMSE. Even frontal executive tests may fail to reveal deficits, as such tests rely more upon dorsolateral prefrontal cortical regions whereas the pathology in FTD involves the orbitomesial frontal cortex. More recently devised tests of decision making and complex planning may be more sensitive. Tasks designed to evaluate so-called 'theory of mind' (see p. 25) and emotion recognition reveal marked problems but remain research-based tools at present.

CT and MRI scans are frequently normal in such patients although volumetric methods of analysis show selective orbitomesial atrophy in the early stages (see Figure 2.3). Functional brain imaging, if available, using SPECT or PET is significantly more sensitive and will usually show frontal hypometabolism.

Semantic dementia

The commonest presentation of this variant of FTD is 'loss of memory for words' and a shrinking vocabulary. Anomia is a salient and very early feature both in spontaneous speech and on confrontational testing. The use of terms such as 'thing' are common and semantically related word substitutions or circumlocutions may occur. Patients often adopt a relatively complex word or phrase which is used repeatedly such as 'situation or special place'. The degree

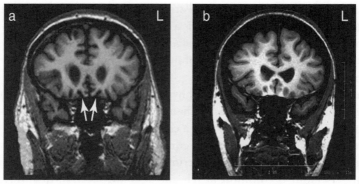

Figure 2.3 Selective atrophy of orbital frontal cortex in patient with early stage behavioural variant frontotemporal dementia.

of comprehension impairment is often masked in conversation due to the clues from context, apparent in phrases such as "how did you get to the hospital today?" However, comprehension of single words, whether written or spoken, is impaired. The feeling of familiarity may remain when the information associated with words has been lost. For instance, when asked the meaning of the word 'hobby' patients often say "hobby, hobby, I'm sure, I should know what that means but I can't remember"; this contrasts with their striking preservation of syntax and phonology. Their difficulty defining the meaning of words initially affects relatively low-familiarity items such as 'harmony, theft, caterpillar, penguin and accordion'. In contrast to Alzheimer's disease, semantic dementia patients show good autobiographical memory for personally experienced events which occurred in the past few years and remain well orientated and attentive.

Category fluency is a sensitive way of detecting semantic deficits with a reduction in the number of examples of animals that can be named. This is even more striking when subjects are asked to name birds or breeds of dog. Repetition is intact, such that patients can repeat multisyllabic words like 'hippopotamus' and 'encyclopaedia' but have no idea of their meaning. Surface dyslexia and surface dysgraphia are typical accompaniments of semantic dementia (see p. 72).

The breakdown in semantic knowledge is most easily demonstrated using verbally based tests but non-verbal tests of associative knowledge (such as the Pyramids and Palm Trees Test) or tasks involving matching sounds-to-pictures, or colouring objects reveal deficits at a very early stage of the disease. The fact that there is breakdown of a central semantic knowledge base has led most authorities to prefer the term semantic dementia rather than progressive fluent aphasia to describe such patients.

In addition to the preservation of episodic memory, visuo-spatial attentional and executive abilities are usually preserved in the early stages which contrast sharply with the typical features of Alzheimer's disease discussed above.

It has become increasingly apparent that many patients with semantic dementia undergo the changes in behaviour similar to those seen in the frontal variant of FTD. Ritualized and obsessive interests such as jigsaws and word searches, alterations in food preference, loss of empathy and emotional coldness are particularly common. As the disease progresses patients may develop Kluver–Bucy syndrome as a result of bilateral damage to the anterior temporal lobe. The features of this syndrome are a tendency to consume inedible things and to put objects in the mouth (hyperorality) and marked alterations in sexual behaviour.

Structural brain imaging (MRI) in patients with semantic dementia reveals atrophy of the polar and inferior temporal regions; the parahippocampal and fusiform gyri are typically affected to the greatest extent with marked asymmetry—the left being worse than the right—sometimes strikingly so (see Figure 2.4). Coronal images are needed to detect these changes in the early stages and CT scans may appear normal due to the angle of acquisition through the temporal lobes.

Over the past decade an increasing number of cases with the much less common pattern of right predominant atrophy have been reported. These patients present with a form of progressive prosopagnosia which, unlike the modality (face)-specific form seen after right occipitotemporal strokes, affects the ability to recognize and identify people regardless of the modality of input (face, name and voice). As in the more typical left predominant semantic dementia cases there is a familiarity effect in that less familiar people (Sean Connery, Gary Lineker) are 'lost' before highly familiar (Tony Blair, David Beckham) famous

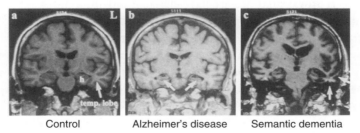

Control   Alzheimer's disease   Semantic dementia

Figure 2.4 Coronal magnetic resonance images in typical cases of Alzheimer's disease and semantic dementia in contrast to a normal age-matched control.

people and family members. Changes in personality are also prominent with the development of coldness and indifference. Strange delusions have also been reported in such cases.

Progressive non-fluent aphasia

In contrast to semantic dementia there is profound disruption of speech output with phonological and grammatical errors. Speech is hesitant and distorted with a typically slowed rate of production. The language syndrome resembles Broca's aphasia in the context of inferior frontal and insula damage. Comprehension of word meaning is preserved and patients perform normally on conceptual and associative tasks such as the Pyramids and Palm Trees Test. The anomia is less profound than in semantic dementia but, in common with this syndrome, there is a marked reduction in fluency affecting both letter- and category-based fluency. Patients show deficits on tests of syntactic comprehension. They have great difficulty repeating multisyllabic words and phrases but retain meaning and hence show the opposite pathology to that seen in semantic dementia.

In common with semantic dementia, episodic memory and visuo-spatial function is well preserved; however, executive deficits are quite common. Behavioural changes seem relatively rare in the early stages. As the disease evolves, oral, orobuccal or limb apraxia commonly develops and there is increasing awareness of the overlap between progressive non-fluent aphasia and CBD.

Imaging studies in progressive non-fluent aphasia show left hemisphere atrophy particularly involving the anterior insula. These changes are easily missed on MRI even with good-quality coronal images. Functional scans [SPECT or fluorodeoxyglucose (FDG)-PET] show more extensive areas of hypometabolism involving the left frontal area.

Vascular dementia

This term has replaced the older label 'multi-infarct dementia' with the realization that only a proportion of patients with cognitive impairment in the context of cerebrovascular disease have classic multi-infarct disease (MID). Patients with MID typically present following a recent large vessel and/or lacunar stroke in the context of thromboembolism from extracranial arteries or small-vessel disease in the brain. Vascular risk factors, especially hypertension, are readily apparent, and many patients have other evidence of atheromatous vascular disease (angina, claudication, cervical bruits, etc.). There may be a stepwise progression, with periods of deterioration followed by more stable periods. Cognitively, impaired attention and frontal features predominate, owing to a concentration of small vascular lesions (lacunes) in the basal ganglia and thalamic regions; but features of cortical dysfunction are also frequently present.

Fluctuations in performance and night-time confusion are very common. Emotional lability, pseudobulbar palsy, gait disturbance and incontinence are characteristic.

The majority of cases with vascular dementia do not have typical MID but instead present with more insidious decline largely indistinguishable from Alzheimer's disease in the context of chronic vascular risk factors with, or without, periods of confusion. MRI imaging reveals diffuse and often confluent white matter pathology involving the periventricular zone and deep white matter (leucoaryosis) as a consequence of occlusion of deep penetrating blood vessels. In contrast to AD, the episodic memory deficit is less dense and involves recall more than retrieval. Patients are slowed up and show gross deficits on executive tasks that require mental flexibility, shifting and response inhibition (such as the Wisconsin Card Sorting Test and the Stroop). Impairments in visuo-spatial and perceptual abilities may be prominent. The majority are apathetic with limited insight.

A diagnosis of vascular dementia should lead to a search for underlying aetiologies including cardiac emboli, thromboembolic atherosclerotic large-vessel disease, vasculitides, prothrombotic states, notably the antiphospholipid syndrome, and, in younger patients with a positive family history of genetic disorders, cerebral autosomal dominant arteriopathy with subcortical infarcts and leucoencephalopathy (CADSIL) or the mitochrondial cytopathies.

Huntington's disease

This genetic disorder is inherited in an autosomal dominant pattern, and has a negligible new mutation rate. Patients have mutations of the Huntington gene on chromosome 3 due to an excess of CAG repeats. The size of the mutation defines the age of onset. Most, but not all, cases occur in the context of a known family history. In apparently *de novo* cases, it is necessary to question several family members to search for clues, such as a family history of psychiatric illness, suicide, dementia, or movement disorders.

Huntington's disease may present with psychiatric, neuropsychological, or neurological symptoms. The peak age of presentation is in the 40s, but the age of presentation can be as late as 70 years. Depression is common; but a schizophrenic-like state with paranoid delusions may also occur. An insidious change in personality, with the development of sociopathic behaviour, is very characteristic. Suicide is a frequent cause of death. The neuropsychological picture is one of subcortical dementia, with marked impairment on tests of attention and frontal function. Patients are forgetful because of impaired attention, but do not show marked amnesia. Language is preserved until late in the course. Visuo-perceptual deficits also occur fairly consistently.

The earliest sign of the movement disorder is a restless fidgetiness of the limbs, which the patient may learn to disguise. Eventually the chorea affects the face and extremities. The gait becomes unsteady and reeling. On walking, characteristic finger-flicking movements may be observed.

Dementia with Lewy bodies

Patients with Parkinson's disease (PD) have Lewy bodies (α-synuclein and ubiquitin-positive inclusions) confined to the substantia nigra and causing dopaminergic depletion. In dementia with Lewy bodies (DLB) these inclusions are more widespread and involve cortical regions as well as the substantia nigra. It is now thought that DLB is as common as vascular dementia in the elderly, and second only to Alzheimer's disease (AD) in terms of neurodegenerative disorders. The clinical features can be considered a hybrid of Parkinson's and AD. Some patients present primarily with parkinsonism often without tremor, others present with progressive cognitive impairment as the prominent feature and develop rigidity and/or bradyphrenia later. Spontaneous fluctuations with periods of frank delirium are characteristic, as are unprovoked visual hallucinations consisting often of people, faces or animals. A history of vivid dreams or even 'acting out' of dreams, so-called REM behavioural sleep disorder, is also common and may precede other features by a number of years. Some patients have falls. Mood disturbance is common and the patients are exquisitely sensitive to small doses of neuroleptics which may precipitate the malignant neuroleptic syndrome (coma, catatonia, hyperpyrexia, hypercatabolism and renal failure).

Cognitively, amnesia is less dense than in AD, but attention and visuospatial/perceptual abilities are typically more impaired. MRI changes in DLB are indistinguishable from AD but SPECT scanning may show disproportionately severe occipital hypoperfusion.

Progressive supranuclear palsy (PSP)

Previously regarded as a very rare parkinsonian syndrome, PSP (or Steele–Richardson–Olszewski syndrome) is now known to be a relatively common disorder which often presents with prominent frontal-executive dysfunction and/or apathy. A reduction of speech output without frank linguistic deficits (so-called dynamic aphasia) is characteristic often with alterations in speech pitch or clarity. Later, frank bulbar features occur. Falls and postural instability are early motor features. Axial rigidity and paralysis of vertical eye movements are characteristic: patients are unable to initiate saccadic (fast) eye movements and later show poor following movements although oculocephalic reflexes (demonstrated by asking the patient to fixate on an object while moving the head) are intact, giving rise to the term 'supranuclear' gaze palsy. The dementia is classically subcortical and progresses fairly rapidly.

Pseudodementia

This term has been used to describe two rather distinct clinical syndromes: hysterical pseudodementia and depressive pseudodementia. The latter is more common, and is undoubtedly the most important treatable cause of memory failure.

Patients with **hysterical pseudodementia** usually present with a fairly abrupt onset of memory and intellectual loss. They typically appear unconcerned. Unlike organic amnesic disorders, the memory impairment is often worse for very salient personal and early-life events. Loss of personal identity may be seen. Memory is strikingly worse when being tested than during informal conversation about recent events. There is usually an identifiable precipitant (such as bereavement, marital problems, or offending) and a past psychiatric history. Patients may show features of the so-called **Ganser's syndrome**, the core symptom of which is the giving of 'approximate answers'. For example, when asked "How many legs does a cow have?", they answer "Three", or in response to "What is two plus two?" they reply "Five". Another classic question is "What colour is an orange?"! As in other hysterical conversion states, there may be an underlying organic disorder that has been grossly exaggerated at either a conscious or a subconscious level.

Depressive pseudodementia is, on the whole, a condition of the elderly. Patients present complaining of poor memory or concentration, and deny overt depression. Clues to the diagnosis are biological features of depression, especially disturbed sleeping, low energy, psychomotor retardation, pessimistic and ruminative thoughts, and a lack of interest in activities and hobbies. The onset of the memory failure is usually relatively acute or subacute. A past or family history of affective illness may be an important marker. On bedside cognitive testing, attention is impaired, and performance on memory and executive tasks is patchy and often inconsistent. Typically, digit span and registration of a name and address are poor, but with repeated trials these improve; and there is not the rapid forgetting of information seen in Alzheimer's disease. Responses on memory and other cognitive tests are frequently "Don't know". Language output is often slow and sparse, but paraphasic errors are not seen. Naming may elicit "Don't know" responses rather than other types of error. In some cases, however, it may be impossible to distinguish true dementia from pseudodementia on simple cognitive tests. If *any* of the above symptoms or signs are present, a psychiatric opinion and a formal neuropsychological evaluation must be sought.

Rapidly progressive dementia

In patients with a history of relatively abrupt onset and progression the differential diagnosis is different to that of typical insidiously progressive dementia. Such patients require intensive investigation to exclude the causes listed in Table 2.8.

Table 2.8 Causes of a rapidly progressive dementing illness

Inflammatory	Cerebral vasculitis
	Multiple sclerosis
	Sarcoidosis
Neoplastic	Primary CNS tumour
	Cerebral metastases
	Paraneoplastic (limbic encephalitis)
Nutritional	Thiamine deficiency (Wernicke–Korsakoff syndrome)
Infectious	Cerebral abscess
	Herpes encephalitis
	Progressive multifocal leukoencephalopathy
	Human immunodeficiency virus
	Subacute sclerosing panencephalitis
	Whipple's disease
Prion	Creutzfeldt–Jakob disease
Vascular	Multiple infarcts (e.g. emboli secondary to endocarditis)
	CADASIL

Imaging in the dementias

The goals of imaging are:

◆ Detecting potentially reversible causes of dementia

◆ Detecting and assessing cerebrovascular disease

◆ Improving the early diagnosis of neurodegenerative diseases, particularly Alzheimer's disease by quantification of atrophy

◆ Indentifying rare but untreatable disorders with distinctive neuroimaging signatures (e.g. leucodystrophies, CADASIL, variant Creutzfeldt–Jakob disease, limbic encephalitis etc.)

After the introduction of CT scanning, a number of studies were undertaken which attempted to develop criteria for imaging with the primary aim of detecting potentially reversible causes and structural causes (tumours, subdural and normal pressure hydrocephalus). A summary of the most robust

Table 2.9 Proposed criteria for imaging patients with dementia if resources are limited

1. Recent onset
2. Age <65 years
3. Fluctuations
4. Focal symptoms or signs
5. History of headache
6. Papilloedema or field defects
7. History of malignancy or head injury
8. Seizures
9. History of stroke or transient ischaemic attack(s)
10. Incontinence
11. Gait ataxia or apraxia

criteria are shown in Table 2.9. Patients with *any* of these features should be scanned. In old-age psychiatric or geriatric practice between 1 and 8% of patients are said to have a potentially reversible cause and about 80% of these will be detected by the strict application of these criteria. Many clinicians would regard this as an unacceptably low rate of detection and would therefore advocate CT or MRI imaging for all patients with dementia.

Young-onset dementia

Over the age of 70 years, three disorders together account for at least 80% of all cases: Alzheimer's disease, dementia with Lewy bodies and vascular dementia, while potentially reversible disorders cause, at most, 5%. Under 60 years of age, the situation is quite different. Alzheimer's disease is still the commonest single cause (30–40%), with frontotemporal dementia running a close second. Vascular dementia and Huntington's disease are also relatively common. This leaves, however, a third of cases due to the other causes shown in Table 2.3, some of which are treatable, while many are genetically determined. The basic message is that rare disorders together account for a sizeable proportion of early-onset cases and the younger the patient the more likely you are to find an unusual disease. All patients aged <60 years, or maybe <70 years, require detailed investigation.

Differential Diagnosis of Delirium and Dementia

See Table 2.10 for the features used in the differential diagnosis of delirium and dementia.

Table 2.10 Differential diagnosis of delirium and dementia

Feature	Delirium	Dementia
Onset	Acute, often at night	Insidious
Course	Fluctuating, with lucid intervals during the day; worse at night	Stable over the course of the day
Duration	Hours to weeks	Months or years
Awareness	Reduced	Clear
Alertness	Abnormally low or high	Usually normal
Attention	Impaired, causing distractibility; fluctuation over the course of the day	Relatively unaffected; impaired in DLB and vascular dementia
Orientation	Usually impaired for time; tendency to mistake unfamiliar places and persons	Impaired in later stages
Short-term (working) memory	Always impaired	Normal in early stages
Episodic memory	Impaired	Impaired
Thinking	Disorganized, delusional	Impoverished
Perception	Illusions and hallucinations, usually visual and common	Absent in earlier stages, common later; common in DLB
Speech	Incoherent, hesitant, slow or rapid	Difficulty in finding words
Sleep–wake cycle	Always disrupted	Usually normal

DLB, dementia with Lewy bodies.

Chapter 3

Localized Cognitive Functions

The functions ascribed to the dominant, usually left, cerebral hemisphere show much more clear-cut laterality than those associated with the so-called 'minor hemisphere'. This applies particularly to spoken language. Since language is such an important component of human cognition, and aphasia frequently complicates both focal and diffuse degenerative brain disease, I have dedicated a large section to discussing aspects of normal and abnormal language function. There then follows a brief description of disorders of calculation (acalculia) and of higher-order motor control (apraxia).

The second half of the chapter deals with disturbed right hemisphere functions: neglect phenomena, dressing and constructional apraxia, and complex visuo-perceptual deficits (agnosias).

Localized cognitive functions can be summarized as follows:

A. Dominant hemisphere

- Spoken language—most aspects of spoken language (phonology, syntax, semantics)
- Reading and writing
- Calculation
- Praxis (higher motor control)

B. Non-dominant hemisphere

- Spatially directed attention
- Complex visuo-perceptual skills
- Constructional abilities
- Prosodic components of language (tone, melody, intonation)
- Emotional processing (see Chapter 1)

Language

The general outline of this section is as follows.

- Definitions and causes of aphasia and mutism
- Cerebral dominance, aspects of applied anatomy, and the role of the minor right hemisphere
- Neurolinguistics made simple: a brief coverage of phonology, syntax and semantics, plus the dual-route hypothesis of reading and writing
- The principles of classifying aphasic syndromes
- A description of the commoner syndromes: Broca's, Wernicke's, transcortical motor and sensory, and anomic aphasia
- Disorders of reading: the dyslexias
- Disorders of writing: the dysgraphias

Aphasia

Aphasia is defined as a loss or impairment of language function caused by brain damage. Language should be separated from speech, since the two may be damaged independently. Speech is the term applied to co-ordinated muscle activity for oral communication and to the neural control of this activity; language is the complex symbolic signal system used by individuals to communicate with one another. Clearly language is not only a spoken system, as communication occurs by reading and writing, and these functions may break down independently, to produce alexia or agraphia,* respectively. Language disorders may also be observed in the congenitally mute who use sign language.

Disturbances of articulatory processes arise from a variety of pathologies involving peripheral speech mechanisms, as in bulbar palsy, and in cerebellar and basal ganglia deficits. Dysarthria frequently accompanies acute anterior left hemisphere lesions, but may also occur with acute right-sided lesions. Thus dysarthria and aphasia may coexist, but one is often seen without the other. Mutism is a complete failure of speech output which, if acquired, usually signifies either a severe language disorder or an articulation disorder, although occasionally mutism may be seen in psychiatrically ill patients (catatonia or hysteria).

---

* The terms aphasia and dysphasia are used interchangeably, although technically aphasia should mean loss of language function and dysphasia should refer to a disturbance of language. The same applies to the terms alexia and dyslexia, and to the terms agraphia and dysgraphia).

Causes of aphasia

Focal lesions

- Strokes, usually middle cerebral artery territory infarcts or haemorrhages
- Tumours, either intrinsic (for example, gliomas, metastases) or extrinsic (for example meningiomas)
- Trauma
- Abscess
- Other space-occupying lesions, tuberculomas, etc.

Dementias

- Alzheimer's disease
- Frontotemporal lobar degeneration (Pick's disease) (see p. 42): semantic dementia, progressive non-fluent aphasia; however, note that dementias rarely cause classical aphasic syndromes

Causes of mutism

Strokes

- Acute global aphasia (middle cerebral artery strokes) accompanied by severely impaired comprehension, reading and writing
- Acute Broca's aphasia: comprehension relatively normal, writing may be unaffected

Disorder of articulation: language and writing normal

- Bulbar palsy (lower motor neuron)
- Pseudobulbar palsy (upper motor neuron)

Psychiatric disorders

- Catanonic stupor
- Schizophrenia
- Severe depression
- Hysterical aphonia
- Elective mutism

Cerebral dominance for language

The left hemisphere is strongly dominant for language functions in most humans. Therefore aphasia very rarely complicates right hemisphere damage in individuals who write with their right hand; when this does occur it is referred to as 'crossed aphasia'. The functional dominance has anatomical parallels; the superior part of the temporal lobe, the planum temporale, is consistently larger on the left side. The situation in left-handers is more complicated; left hemisphere dominance in these individuals is commonly stated to be around 50–60%. In fact, most people who do *not* show a strong preference for writing with their right hand are, to some degree, ambidextrous. Commensurate with this, their language functions are more equally divided between the two hemispheres.

Applied anatomy

Within the left hemisphere, the area of supreme importance for language comprehension and production is the posterior superior temporal lobe (Wernicke's area). Deficits in this area consistently produce gross problems with the decoding of spoken and written language, and in the assembly of correct language output with phonological and semantic speech errors. The other major language area is in the inferior frontal lobe (Broca's area) and the adjacent anterior insula. Lesions here produce faltering, non-fluent, and distorted language output, with simplified or disturbed grammatical structure, although the comprehension of spoken and written language is largely intact. The insula is thought to be key for phonological assembly and lesions restricted to this area cause so-called speech apraxia in which patients have great difficulty repeating strings of syllables. The inferior frontal and superior temporal regions are connected by means of the arcuate fasciculus; lesions here classically cause conduction aphasia, although this syndrome most commonly results from damage to the supramarginal gyrus or surrounding areas (see Figure 3.1).

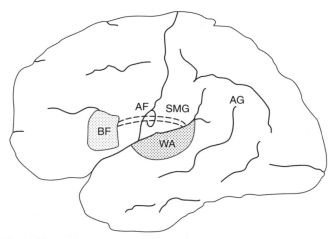

Fig. 3.1 Principal language areas. BA, Broca's area; WA, Wernicke's area; AF, arcuate fasciculus; SMG, supramarginal gyrus; AG, angular gyrus.

One extremely important concept (based in the past on lesion and electro-physiological studies in patients with acquired pathology and, more recently, on functional activation by positron emision tomography (PET) and functional magnetic resonance imaging (fMRI) in normal volunteers) is that Wernicke's area acts as the 'gateway' between the amodal semantic or knowledge system and modality-specific language areas. Patients with lesions to Wernicke's area do not lose knowledge about things in the world as evident from their ability to use objects appropriately and perform picture–picture matching tests. Put simply, they know what a fork or stethoscope are when given the item but have lost the ability to map the arbitrary phonemes 'F'_ 'ORK' to that object. This contrasts with the cross-modal loss which occurs in patients with semantic dementia (see p. 45).

The area most associated with writing ability is the angular gyrus, which is the posterior extension of Wernicke's area, and is situated at the junction of the temporal, parietal, and occipital lobes. Lesions that include the angular gyrus area cause Gerstmann's syndrome, consisting of dysgraphia, dyscalculia, right–left disorientation, and a peculiar deficit in recognition of body parts called finger agnosia.

The minor hemisphere and language

The above statements concerning language dominance require some qualifi-cation, since not all aspects of language show such hemispheric specializa-tion (see Table 3.1). It has become apparent from experimental studies of

Table 3.1 Definitions and neural bases of language functions

Language function	Definition	Neural basis
Phonology	Production and comprehension of appropriately sequenced speech sounds (phonemes)	Left superior temporal lobe and anterior insula
Semantics	Assignment of meaning to words and production of linguistically appropriate individual words	Anterior and inferior temporal lobe (representations) and Wernicke's area (mapping)
Syntax	Assembly of strings of words into sentences using pronouns, prepositions, tenses, etc.	Broca's area
Prosody	(i) Fine tuning by intonation, stress, cadence, etc. (ii) Emotional expression	Left anterior hemisphere, basal ganglia Right hemisphere

split-brain subjects (i.e. studies following corpus collosal section for intractable epilepsy) that, even in right-handers, the right hemisphere has a considerable capacity for understanding simple words, especially nouns, although it is unable to utilize the apparatus of speech for responding. This limited ability of the non-dominant hemisphere may explain some of the recovery seen even after devastating left hemisphere damage with resultant global aphasia. Also notable is the right hemisphere's role in some non-linguistic aspects of language expression and comprehension. Although the linguistic components—phonology, syntax and semantics—convey the principal meaning of language (see below), there are in addition more subtle modulations which we use to imply attitude and emotion. These features have been termed **prosody**, which refers to the melody, pauses, intonation, stresses and accents that enhance and enliven speech. Severely dysprosodic speech occurs with anterior left hemisphere damage. More subtle deficits in conveying and interpreting the emotion or affective components of language consistently accompany right-handed lesions—so-called 'emotional dysprosody'. This is interesting in the context of other non-language-based specialization of the minor hemisphere. Patients with right hemisphere damage may show impairment on emotional judgement tasks involving faces.

Neurolinguistics made simple

True aphasia results from the breakdown in the linguistic components of language. These can be divided into phonological, semantic (or lexical) and syntactic aspects.

Phonology This is the term applied to the sound pattern of human language. The smallest segment of spoken language is the phoneme, which is more or less the same as the sound represented by a single letter in alphabetic writing systems, such as the sounds represented by the letter 'k' in 'kiss' or the letters 'sh' in 'should'. Each language consists of a finite number of phonemes, which can be ordered to produce an almost infinite number of words. They can therefore be considered the building-blocks of language. Patients may be impaired in the ability to organize phonemes in sequence, which results in phonemic (or literal) paraphasias, which may be real-word approximations (SITTER for SISTER; STALE for SNAIL, etc.) or neologisms (FENCIL for PENCIL; POOT for SUIT; BORINGE for ORANGE). Phonemic decoding (necessary for distinguishing PEAR from BEAR, or FIT from BIT) is clearly critical for language comprehension. Both phonemic production and decoding depend on the superior temporal region. Most patients with middle cerebral artery strokes and aphasia have some deficit in phonological processing.

Semantics The term semantics denotes the referential meaning of words. The fact that we know the correct meanings of 'aunt', 'uncle', 'sister', etc., and that 'canary' refers to a small yellow bird, depends on our ability to map this arbitrary sound pattern into the underlying conceptual representation. This process can break down in two ways: a problem with the mapping process (as in Wernicke's aphasia) or a loss of the representation (as in semantic dementia). Our store of words is sometimes called the 'mental lexicon'; but semantics refers to more than a simple store of word forms—it encompasses our fund of knowledge of the world. This is discussed more fully in the section on semantic memory (see p. 19). Breakdown within the semantic system results in a failure to understand the referential meaning of words, so that on naming or in spontaneous speech, paraphasias (ORANGE for APPLE, SISTER for BROTHER, etc.) or superordinate substitutions (ANIMAL for GIRAFFE) are produced. Mere failure to access the correct word in the lexicon typically produces word-finding difficulty, with abrupt cut-offs in speech or circumlocutions ["it's that thin green vegetable that you eat with your fingers" (asparagus)]. Comprehension clearly depends on the accurate assignment of meaning to heard words. A breakdown in this process impairs single-word comprehension. The dominant temporal lobe plays a key role in lexico-semantic processes. Contemporary neuroimaging studies indicate that the superior temporal region (Wernicke's area), the basal temporal areas (areas 20 and 35) and the angular gyrus (area 37) form a complex network, with Wernicke's area being the central co-ordinating region.

Syntax Words are strung together to form phrases or sentences in a complex way that obeys strict grammatical rules. The correct use of these non-substantive components of language—articles, prepositions, pronouns, adverbs, verb endings, etc.—is referred to as syntax. A reduction or loss of syntactic production, agrammatism, is found in patients with Broca's type aphasia. The production of sentences with incorrect use of these syntactic elements, termed paragrammatism, is a feature of Wernicke's aphasia. Disorders of comprehension affecting predominately the syntactic aspects of language can also be demonstrated in patients with damage to the inferior frontal lobe and in the dementias.

Each of these components of language—phonology, syntax, and semantics—can be independently damaged. Furthermore, the deficit may involve input, output, or both. Since the neural circuits underlying these processes function in parallel and overlap anatomically, focal lesions invariably produce complex deficits. Many neurolinguists would argue that no two aphasia patients are exactly alike; but, luckily for clinicians, recognizable clinical syndromes usually emerge, at least after the phase of acute damage. It is worth emphasizing the point that the classical descriptions of the aphasic syndromes (Broca's, Wernicke's and conduction aphasia, etc.) were based on chronic stable brain lesions. It is often difficult to apply this classification to acute stroke patients, the majority of whom have either a global aphasia or an atypical unclassifiable aphasia. Similarly, patients with language breakdown secondary to progressive degenerative brain disease, such as Alzheimer's or frontotemporal dementia, do not develop classical aphasic syndromes. For these reasons, analysis of language disturbance is best considered in terms of the linguistic components outlined above.

Theories of reading and writing

A similar linguistic analysis can be applied to disorders of reading and writing. In the case of writing, phonology becomes orthography (or spelling). In this respect, it is important to remember that the rules of English orthography are complex, with many unique exceptions. By knowing the rules of English pronunciation it is possible to read and spell many words correctly (HINT, GLINT; GAVE, BRAVE; CASE, BASE; etc.) and plausible non-words (NEG, GLEM, GORTH, etc.); but not words with irregular spelling-to-sound correspondence (for instance, PINT; HAVE; ISLAND; YACHT). Clearly such irregular or exceptional words cannot be read *or* spelt correctly by applying spelling-to-sound rules, but rather must be pronounced or spelt by directly accessing word-specific knowledge about their phonology and orthography. The evidence from patients with acquired dyslexia has been used to argue that there are two parallel systems for reading and writing; one utilizes a sound-based route for reading and writing, and the other uses the more direct meaning route (see Figure 3.2). These systems can break down independently, to produce different types of dyslexia and dysgraphia, which are described below. An alternative view is based upon computational interactive models of cognition. The so-called triangle model proposes that three core processes—semantics, phonology and orthography—interact (Figure 3.3). This system quickly learns to read correctly regular words based on print-to-sound correspondances in the language without the need for semantic support. Irregular words present more difficulty (as anyone with children learning to read and spell English know) and the system has to learn each of these unique word-to-sound mappings. Some irregular words have very frequent occurrence in English (HAVE, ONCE) and are quickly learnt, others are of low frequency (MAUVE, GIST, EPITOME) and are learnt slowly, if ever. For the latter words, semantic support is very important because when semantics break down patients have difficulty pronouncing and spelling low-frequency irregular words (this is termed 'surface dyslexia').

Classifying aphasia syndromes

I have avoided the terms expressive and receptive aphasia, which, in my opinion, are misleading; virtually all aphasic patients have difficulty with language

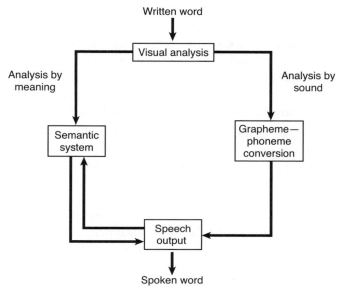

Fig. 3.2 Dual-route model of reading.

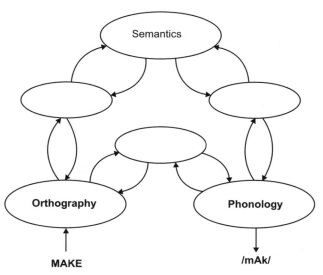

Fig. 3.3 Triangle model based on computational theories.

expression, although the linguistic processes underlying the deficit differ. Patients with left anterior lesions have a disturbance of language output, producing laborious and distorted speech. Posterior lesions produce a fluent language output, with phonemic and semantic paraphasic errors. Both patient groups have problems with 'expression'.

For the purpose of gross clinical diagnosis and clinico-anatomical correlation, four aspects of language should be considered (see Table 3.2).

1. *Fluency*. This aspect divides aphasic syndromes into those related to damage anterior and posterior to the sylvian fissure. Non-fluent speech is slow and laboriously produced, with abnormal speech rhythm and melody, poor articulation, shortened phrase length, and often a preferential use of substantive words (especially nouns and some verbs). Non-fluent speech is invariably associated with lesions anterior to the sylvian fissure. Fluent speech, by contrast, is produced at a normal rate, with preserved speech rhythm and melody, good articulation, and normal phrase length. In fluent dysphasia the lesion is located posterior to the sylvian fissure, in Wernicke's area, or more basal temporal regions.

2. *Repetition*. When repetition is defective the lesion is either in the peri-sylvian area or in the so-called 'zone of language'. The latter is in the territory of the middle cerebral artery, and includes both banks of the sylvian fissure, incorporating Broca's area and the insula cortex anteriorly and Wernicke's area posteriorly—and the arcuate fasciculus between them. Where repetition is well preserved compared with spontaneous speech the lesion has spared these primary language areas and is located cortically or subcortically outside the peri-sylvian region. Syndromes associated with sparing of repetition are termed transcortical—either transcortical motor or transcortical sensory.

Table 3.2 Classification of aphasic syndromes according to four parameters

Type of aphasia	Fluency	Repetition	Comprehension	Naming
Global	Non-fluent	✗	✗	✗
Broca's	Non-fluent	✗	✓	✗
Transcortical motor	Non-fluent	✓	✓	✗
Wernicke's	Fluent	✗	✗	✗
Transcortical sensory	Fluent	✓	✗	✗
Conduction	Fluent	✗	✓	✗
Anomic	Fluent	✓	✓	✗

✗, affected; ✓, relatively spared.

3. *Comprehension.* Virtually all dysphasic patients will show some degree of comprehension deficit if tests of syntactic comprehension are used. However, for clinical purposes patients can be readily divided into those with obvious impairment of spoken language comprehension—invariably associated with a damaged temporal lobe—and those in whom comprehension is spared.

4. *Naming.* The ability to name objects, or drawings of objects, is impaired in all aphasic patients to some degree. The type of error, however, varies, as does the response to cueing, as will be described below.

Common aphasic syndromes: Broca's, Wernicke's Conduction, Transcortical and Anomic

For each of the more common aphasic syndromes I shall describe the nature of the spontaneous speech, performance on tests of naming, repetition, and comprehension, writing and reading, and their anatomical localization.

Broca's aphasia In the fully developed syndrome, speech output has two principal characteristics—it is non-fluent and agrammatic—although these two features can dissociate. Typically, there is impairment of word initiation and phoneme selection. This results in slow, effortful, and laboured speech, which is distorted with frequent word approximations (phonemic paraphasias). Attempts at word or sentence repetition show the same features. The second major component of spontaneous speech is agrammatism. This is a simplification of grammatical form, with a notable reduction in function words (prepositions, articles, etc.). At its most severe, the patient is restricted to telegraphic utterances. It should be noted that this feature is present only in a minority of cases; most patients with Broca's aphasia manifest only a simplification or reduction in syntactic complexity rather than an absolute loss.

Naming on confrontation is impaired, but the patient often responds when a phonemic cue (the beginning sound of the word) is provided, and is able to choose the correct name from amongst a number of alternatives. Auditory comprehension, although typically preserved in ordinary conversation, may break down when it is studied by using syntactically complex commands ('touch the book after touching the pen'). The written output of patients with Broca's aphasia mirrors their spoken language. It is characterized by misspellings, letter omissions, perseverations, and agrammatic sentences. Reading aloud is disturbed. On single-word reading, the syndrome of deep dyslexia (see p. 72) may occur, in which subjects make frequent semantic errors (SISTER for UNCLE; PARROT for CANARY, etc.), and are unable to read small function words, or unfamiliar, phonologically plausible non-words (CHOG, LAVE, GORTH).

Anatomical localization. The term 'Broca's aphasia' has become more descriptive than anatomical. Neuroimaging studies have shown that lesions purely restricted to Broca's area (the inferior frontal lobe) produce a transient disturbance in speech output, not the other features of Broca's aphasia. The symptom complex of Broca's aphasia occurs after more extensive damage to the frontoparietal region, corresponding to the area supplied by the anterior branch of the middle cerebral artery. Moreover, the fully developed syndrome is rarely encountered in acute stroke patients, but evolves over time from a more global aphasic syndrome. A variant of Broca's aphasia, known as **speech apraxia**, is seen in association with anterior insula damage. In such patients there is disintegration of speech output and they have inordinate difficulty repeating multisyllabic words (e.g. caterpillar) and sequences of syllables (PA … TA … KA) leading to multiple approximation attempts. Some patients with progressive non-fluent aphasia have classic features of speech apraxia.

Wernicke's aphasia In Wernicke's aphasia, spontaneous speech is fluent and paraphasic. In the acute stages speech output often consists of strings of phonemic and semantic paraphasias and their combinations, sometimes producing neologistic jargon. In contrast to Broca's aphasia, there is little effort in speaking, and no dysarthria. Indeed, in many cases there is an increased speech production rate, with a tendency to acceleration. Melody and intonation are preserved. It would therefore be impossible to detect Wernicke's aphasia in a patient speaking a language unfamiliar to the examiner. There is relative preservation of grammatical structure, but speech lacks information-conveying nouns and verbs ('Yes, I should say so', 'I mean', 'I'm a redax', 'no toxicat', 'that is to say …', 'you know what I mean', etc.). Often abnormal syntactic inflections are produced; this is termed paragrammatism. Patients are usually unaware of their communication problem. Naming is severely impaired; patients often produce phonemic or semantic errors, but are not aided by phonemic cues, and are typically unable to select the correct name when offered a choice by the examiner.

Auditory comprehension is always impaired. In severe cases, patients are unable to point on command to common objects in an array (for example, 'point to the keys'); but simple body commands may be preserved. Linguistically, patients have difficulty with phoneme discrimination, and with assigning mapping strings of phonemes to their internal semantic representation.

The comprehension of written text is usually similar to auditory comprehension. However, some patients have superior reading ability, perhaps in association with relative sparing of more anteriorly placed parts of the superior temporal lobe. When writing, letters are well formed, but patients produce aphasic, disjointed, and repetitive text, containing few nouns and verbs.

Anatomical localization. Unlike Broca's aphasia, Wernicke's aphasia correlates fairly well with destruction of Wernicke's area. Right-handed patients with the full-blown syndrome of fluent, paraphasic and paragrammatic speech and severe impairment of auditory comprehension almost invariably have suffered damage to the posterior superior temporal lobe of the left cerebral hemisphere. The extent of the comprehension deficit and the prognosis for recovery depends on the degree of damage to Wernicke's area.

Conduction aphasia Named after damage to the main conducting tract (arcuate fasciculus) joining Broca's and Wernicke's areas, conduction aphasia is characterized by fluent but paraphasic speech. The paraphasias are mainly phonemic (for instance SITTER for SISTER; FENCIL for PENCIL). In contrast to Wernicke's aphasia, comprehension of speech and written material is much better. Repetition is highly abnormal; patients typically produce strings of phonemic approximations in an attempt to repeat a phrase, termed *conduit d'approche* (ROY ARTCRY … ROYIT ARTIL … ROYOT ARTIMERY, etc.). Digit span is characteristically very limited. There is almost always anomia because of multiple phonemic paraphasic errors. Reading aloud parallels the performance of repetition; but comprehension of silent reading may be very good.

Anatomical localization. The traditional locus of pathology in conduction aphasia has been in the supramarginal gyrus, i.e. the gyrus lying above and around the posterior end of the sylvian fissure and the adjacent white matter tracts (see Figure 2.1) which thereby separates the temporal from the frontal language areas. Many exceptions to this classic localization have been reported, although most cases have involved lesions round the sylvian fissure. Conduction aphasia most often occurs at a stage of recovery from Wernicke's aphasia. When it occurs as an acute syndrome the prognosis for complete recovery is very good.

Transcortical aphasias Early aphasiologists observed that some patients with aphasia retained competence at repeating language which they did not understand. They postulated the existence of a 'transcortical pathway' directly linking the so-called 'auditory language centre' and the 'verbal motor centre', thus bypassing meaning. The term 'transcortical' has persisted, despite abandonment of the supporting theory, and is now used purely descriptively.

The features common to the transcortical dysphasias are preserved repetition and cortical or deep white matter damage at, or beyond, the periphery of the peri-sylvian language areas.

Transcortical motor aphasia. Transcortical motor aphasia (TMA) shares many similarities with Broca's aphasia: spontaneous language output is very sparse and dysarthric, but with few paraphasic errors. Sentence repetition is, by contrast, strikingly preserved, and comprehension of verbal and written language is very good. Written output parallels spoken output. Lesions responsible for TMA are located in the dominant frontal lobe anterior and superior to Broca's area. This is the type of aphasia typically seen with anterior cerebral artery infarction, and may follow a period of initial muteness. In these cases the critical lesion is in the supplementary motor area in the superomedial parasagittal region of the frontal lobe. TMA may also occur in patients with frontotemporal lobar degeneration (See page 42).

Transcortical sensory aphasia. Transcortical sensory aphasia (TSA) is similar to Wernicke's aphasia, the language output being fluent but contaminated with semantic paraphasic errors. Comprehension is severely defective at the level of linking sound to meaning. However, phonemic processing is intact, and the patient is therefore able to repeat words and long sentences, but cannot extract meaning from language. Reading and writing are similar to those in Wernicke's aphasia. The site of the lesion is said to be in the border zone of the parietotemporal junction, which therefore preserves the primary language areas, but disconnects them from posterior brain areas. A language syndrome akin to TSA occurs in advanced Alzheimer's disease and in patients with the temporal lobe variant of frontotemporal lobar degeneration, better known as semantic dementia. In the latter syndrome the fluent aphasia is simply one manifestation of a more generalized or amodal loss of knowledge (see p. 45).

Anomic aphasia Difficulty in word-finding on confrontational naming tasks is the rule in virtually all aphasic patients. Problems with word access in free conversation producing either abrupt cut-offs in mid-sentence, circumlocutions, or paraphasic substitutions, are also ubiquitous. Only when the severity of naming problems stands out above all other language deficits is the term 'anomic aphasia' used. This is a common syndrome. It is a frequent residual deficit following recovery from one of the other types of aphasia, and is the characteristic language abnormality in the earlier stages of Alzheimer's disease. A space-occupying lesion present anywhere in the dominant hemisphere may manifest as anomic aphasia.

Anomia is, therefore, the least useful localizing sign in aphasia. But the acute onset of pure anomic aphasia suggests a lesion in the left temporoparietal area. When the injury extends to the angular gyrus, alexia and agraphia may appear.

Category-specific anomia. This is the term given to a deficit in naming items of a particular category. A well-documented form of this is colour anomia. Patients have a specific deficit in naming colours on confrontation or in pointing to colours when they are named by others (see p. 91). Other examples of category-specific anomias involve naming living things or non-living things. In the latter syndromes there is loss of general knowledge about the affected category, so that generating definitions, answering questions about semantic features, and comprehending on picture-pointing tests are also impaired. Since these deficits affect more than purely naming, they are more properly considered as disorders of semantic memory (see p. 19). Patients who have sustained temporal lobe damage from *herpes simplex* virus encephalitis seem to be particularly vulnerable to category-specific semantic memory deficits.

It is worth noting at this point that the process of naming, although apparently simple and automatic in normal circumstances, depends upon a complex sequence of processes—visuo-perceptual, semantic, lexical, phonological and articulatory—each of which may be disrupted. Disorders of visuo-perceptual and semantic processing are considered more fully under the heading of visual agnosia (see p. 85).

Formal tests of language (see Appendix for details)

1. Spontaneous language elicited by complex picture description (for example the Beach scene illustrated in Chapter 7 (p. 180) and the famous 'cookie jar theft' picture from the Boston Diagnostic Aphasia Examination).

2. Naming to confrontation of the line-drawings graded in familiarity (for example the Boston Naming Test, Graded Naming Test).

3. Comprehension of increasingly syntactically complex commands (for example The Token Test and the Test for the Reception of Grammar or TROG).

4. Word–picture matching tests of single-word (semantic) comprehension (for example the Peabody Picture Vocabulary Test and the word–picture matching test from the Cambridge Semantic Battery).

5. Aphasia batteries such as the Boston Diagnostic Aphasia Examination (BDAE), the Western Aphasia Battery (WAB), and the Psycholinguistic Assessments of Language Processing in Aphasia (PALPA) all provide a systematic and thorough evaluation of language abilities, but are time-consuming and not generally used in routine clinical neuropsychological practice.

Disorders of Reading—The Dyslexias

Disturbances of reading can be divided into two broad categories: (i) those in which there is a defect in the early visual components of decoding written script, the so-called **peripheral dyslexias**; and (ii) those in which there is a breakdown in the normal linguistic processes involved in deriving meaning from words, the **central dyslexias** (see Table 3.3).

Table 3.3 Types of dyslexia and their localizations

Types of dyslexia	Localization
Peripheral dyslexias	
Preserved oral and written spelling, and ability to identify words spelt aloud	
1. Alexia without agraphia • letter-by-letter reading	Left medial occipital lobe
2. Neglect dyslexia • errors reading left-hand or initial part of words	Right hemisphere lesions
Central linguistic dyslexias	
Linguistically based, invariably affect oral spelling	
1. Surface dyslexia • Breakdown of whole word (lexical) reading • Difficulty with irregularly spelt words • Phonologically plausible errors	Left temporo-parietal region and semantic dementia
2. Deep dyslexia • Loss of sound-based (phonological) reading • Semantic errors • Difficulty with function and abstract words • Inability to read non-words	Extensive left hemisphere lesions
3. Phonological dyslexia • Non-word reading	

Peripheral dyslexias

Alexia without agraphia (pure alexia)

This rare syndrome was important in establishing the concept of internal discon-nection of cortical areas although the theoretical interpretation of pure alexia is now more controversial. In most cases there is an acute inability to comprehend any written material. By contrast, the patient recognizes words spelled aloud. Writing is preserved, but patients are unable to read their own written output. Spoken language is also normal. With time, the ability to read individual letters often returns. When this happens, words are spelled aloud by the patients and recognized auditorily, so that they adopt a 'letter-by-letter' reading strategy. Because of this, there is a marked word-length effect, so that, unlike normals, patients with letter-by-letter reading are very slow at reading longer words. The syndrome is usually accompanied by right homonymous hemianopia.

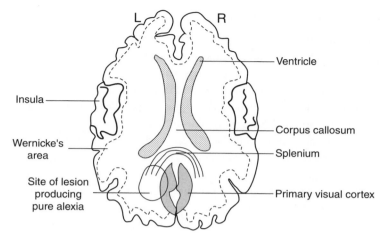

Fig. 3.4 Alexia without agraphia: lesion causes interruption of information flow to the left-sided language areas from ipsilateral and contralateral visual areas (via splenium).

Defects in colour naming (with intact colour vision) or impairment of colour perception (achromatopsia) may also occur (see p. 91). This symptom complex usually accompanies infarction of the medial aspect of the left occipital lobe, often with involvement of the splenium of the corpus callosum, following occlusion of the left posterior cerebral artery (see Figure 3.4). The classic theory for the genesis of alexia without agraphia is as follows: because of the right hemianopia patients cannot read in the right visual field. Words can be seen on the left side, and are therefore projected to the right hemisphere. However, the lesion in the splenium prevents transfer of the visual information from the right to the left side. The primary language areas are spared, but are disconnected from incoming visual information. The strategy adopted of identifying each individual letter is thought to occur initially in the right hemisphere, which then enables access to pronunciation in the left hemisphere. More recently this disconnection has been doubted, rather it has been argued that the infarction damages the so-called 'word form' area which disrupts the ability to process whole words but also single letters to be decoded.

Neglect dyslexia

In neglect dyslexia, which usually complicates right parietal lesions, there is failure to read correctly the left half of words (for example LAND is read for ISLAND; PEACH is read as BEACH, etc.). This syndrome is discussed more fully in the context of other hemineglect phenomena (see p. 79). Neglect dyslexia arising from a left hemisphere lesion and thereby affecting the right half of words is exceptionally rare and difficult to detect.

Central (linguistic) dyslexias

Most aphasic patients have some disturbance of either reading aloud or of comprehension of text. Indeed, this is one of the most sensitive markers of language disturbance, and many patients who have otherwise recovered from acute aphasic syndromes find that they no longer derive pleasure from reading. In the aphasic syndromes, reading aloud usually parallels other oral language abilities. Broca's aphasics have particular difficulty reading grammatical morphemes (function words like OF and AT, and verb inflections such as -ED) and make numerous errors, producing laboured and faltering oral reading. Their comprehension of complex text is usually poor. Most patients with moderate or severe Wernicke's aphasia are severely dyslexic, and make numerous paraphasic errors. Reading is relatively intact in patients with diffuse brain damage and in the early stages of Alzheimer's disease. Since the ability to pronounce irregular words correctly is highly educationally dependent, a test of irregular word reading, the National Adult Reading Test (or NART), is widely used to predict premorbid intellectual ability. Two broad types of linguistically based dyslexic syndrome can be distinguished on single-word reading.

Surface dyslexia

In this form of dyslexia, there is breakdown in the whole-word (lexical) representations, so that reliance is placed on sub-word correspondences between letters and sounds (the so-called grapheme–phoneme conversion system). This use of the 'surface' features produces few problems reading words with regular sound-to-spelling correspondence. But errors occur when attempting to read words which deviate from the typical pattern of spelling-to-sound correspondence in English, so-called exception words (PINT, ISLAND, MAUVE, etc.). The most frequent mistake is to produce regularization error (PINT to rhyme with MINT). There is usually a marked frequency effect, so that the ability to read low-frequency irregular words is most affected. As well as occurring with posteriorly placed left temporo-parietal strokes, this syndrome is almost universal in semantic dementia and in other patients with breakdown in the semantic system. The theory advanced to explain surface dyslexia as described on p. 62.

Deep dyslexia

This extremely rare syndrome is characterized by an inability to translate orthography to phonology, which means that patients with this disorder are required to read entirely via meaning. They are completely unable to read plausible nonwords such as NEG, GLEM, GORTH etc. The cardinal symptom which is likely to bring attention to deep dyslexia is the semantic error: when trying to read single words aloud, the patient produces responses related in meaning (but not sound) to the target (for example, reading CANARY as PARROT; TULIP as CROCUS; SISTER as UNCLE, etc.). Visual errors are also common (for example, SWORD for WORDS, SCANDAL for SANDALS). There is usually great difficulty in reading small function words (IS, OF, AND, THE, etc.), and a relative impairment in reading abstract compared with concrete words. Most patients with deep dyslexia have suffered extensive left hemisphere damage. Opinions are divided as to whether the features of deep dyslexia result from the residual malfunctioning left hemisphere, or from the right hemisphere's attempt at reading. The latter gains support from the characteristics of right hemisphere reading in split-brain patients, which resemble in many ways the features of deep dyslexia.

Phonological dyslexia

Phonological dyslexia is a rare form of dyslexia that affects mainly the ability to read non-words.

Tests of reading ability (see Chapter 5 for details)

1. Text reading.
2. Single-word reading using words with regular and exceptional spelling-to-sound correspondence (such as the National Adult Reading Test, NART), and plausible non-words.
3. Single-letter identification.

Disorders of Writing—The Dysgraphias

The production of well-formed and linguistically correct, flowing script depends upon the integration of motor control, visuo-spatial and kinaesthetic functions, and the symbolic aspects of the language system. It is not surprising, therefore, that writing abilities are fragile, and that brain dysfunction of very varied types produces dysgraphia. Dysgraphia is more prominent than dyslexia in patients with degenerative brain disease. It is a striking early feature in corticobasal degeneration. Three main varieties of writing disturbance can be identified (see Table 3.4).

Dyspraxic dysgraphia

Writing disturbance is said to have a dyspraxic quality if there is a disturbance in the smooth automatic production of written elements due to a breakdown in motor control. Letters may be inverted or reversed, and are often illegible. Copying is also abnormal. Oral spelling is preserved. Dyspraxic dysgraphia

Table 3.4 Types of dysgraphia and their localizations

Types of dysgraphia	Localization
Dyspraxic dysgraphia	
Oral spelling intact, defective copying	Dominant parietal or frontal lobe
Neglect dysgraphia	
Wide left margin or mis-spelling of initial part of words. Other neglect phenomena present	Right hemisphere lesions
Central (linguistic) dysgraphias	
Written oral spelling affected	
1. Lexical (surface) dysgraphia • Breakdown of lexical route for spelling • Difficult spelling irregular words • Phonologically plausible errors	Left temporo-parietal region and semantic dementia
2. Deep dysgraphia • Breakdown of sound-based route for spelling • Semantic errors • Unable to spell non-words • Better concrete than abstract spelling	Extensive left hemisphere damage
3. Phonological dysgraphia • As above, but without semantic errors	Unknown

most often accompanies dominant parietal lobe damage, and features of ideo-motor limb dyspraxia are usually present. Dominant frontal lobe lesions may occasionally produce pure dyspraxic dysgraphia.

Spatial or neglect dysgraphia

This disorder of writing usually accompanies non-dominant hemisphere lesions. It can be easily differentiated from the other dysgraphias because of the invariable association with other visuo-spatial and perceptual abnormalities (spatial neglect, drawing problems, etc.), and by the characteristics of the writing: a wide left margin and a tendency to miss out, or mis-spell, the first few letters of individual words (RUSH for BRUSH; DOY for JOY, etc.).

Central (linguistic) dysgraphias

These almost always accompany some degree of spoken language disturbance or dyslexia. The pattern of deficit tends to parallel the accompanying aphasia. Anteriorly placed dominant hemisphere lesions produce slow, effortful writing which is poorly formed, with mis-spellings, omissions, reversals and perse-verations. Agrammatism may also be observed. Patients with Wernicke's aphasia may have preserved motor aspects of handwriting ability, but produce paraphasic errors and show word-finding impairments. Difficulty spelling and writing is a common early feature of corticobasal degeneration.

In parallel with the central dyslexias, two broad types of linguistic dysgraphia can be distinguished.

Lexical (surface) dysgraphia

The lexical (semantic) system uses whole-word retrieval by consulting internal memory stores of known spellings. This system is important for spelling familiar but orthographically irregular words (for example, CHOIR, PINT, ISLAND, NAIVE) and homophones (words with the same pronunciation but different spelling, for example ATE—EIGHT). Damage to this system produces a lexical agraphia characterized by particular problems in spelling irregular words and the production of errors that are phonologically plausible (MENIS for MENACE, COFF for COUGH, etc.). This syndrome has been described in patients with lesions in rather diverse sites in the left temporoparietal region. It is also a fairly consistent finding in patients with advanced Alzheimer's disease and with semantic dementia in whom there is a breakdown of the semantic system (see p 45).

Deep dysgraphia

The alternative, phonological, spelling system uses sound–letter (phoneme–grapheme) rules. Disruption of this system produces phonological agraphia, in which patients are unable to spell unfamiliar words and non-words (for example VIB, CHOG, LAVE).

Deep dysgraphia results from more profound breakdown in the sound-based spelling route, with additional damage to the semantic system. As in deep dyslexia, semantic errors occur (SISTER for AUNT; SKY for SUN), and there is a strong effect of word class, in that those affected are better at spelling concrete than abstract words. Most patients with this syndrome have suffered extensive left hemisphere damage.

Phonological dysgraphia

In the majority of patients with linguistically based dysgraphias, oral and written spelling are equally impaired. As a general rule, disturbed writing with spared oral spelling suggests a dyspraxic or neglect dysgraphia.

Tests of writing ability (see Chapter 5 for details)

1. Spontaneous writing of sentences.
2. Writing words with regular and exceptional spelling-to-sound correspondence and plausible non-words.
3. Copying words and single letters.

Syndromes of Calculating Impairment

Acalculia, anarithmetria, spatial dyscalculia

Acalculia, a disturbance in the ability to comprehend or write numbers properly, is common in patients with aphasia; but rare instances where number and language abilities dissociate have been reported. The angular gyrus region in the left hemisphere appears to be important for numeracy. A separate disorder, **anarithmetria**, is characterized by the inability to perform number manipulations. Patients with this disorder correctly recognize and reproduce individual numbers and know their values, but cannot perform computations (addition, subtraction, etc.). This disorder is relatively common in patients with dementias, particularly Alzheimer's disease. A third cause of difficulty performing written calculations is so-called **spatial dyscalculia**. This syndrome, in which patients have difficulty aligning columns of figures and performing carrying tasks, complicates right hemisphere damage, and is invariably associated with other neglect phenomena.

Gerstmann's syndorme

This rare symptom complex is also referred to as the **angular gyrus syndrome**, because of the localization of the causative lesions. The features are:

1. Agraphia of the central (or linguistic) type.
2. Acalculia, producing difficulty with number reading, number writing, or calculations.
3. Right–left disorientation, by which is meant a disorder in demonstrating the correct hand (or other body part) to command.
4. Finger agnosia, a term applied to deficits ranging from the inability to name the fingers to inability to point or move a finger when its name is given. A more subtle indicator of this can be a difficulty in locating the fingers(s) touched by the examiner.

Since these features can occur in isolation or in any combination the usefulness of this syndrome in clinical practice is rather questionable.

Disorders of Praxis—The Apraxias

Apraxia is the inability to carry out complex motor acts despite intact motor and sensory systems and co-ordination, good comprehension, and full co-operation. The term 'apraxia' should be applied only to deficits with a motoric basis. Several unrelated disorders use the same term (dressing apraxia, construction apraxia, verbal apraxia of speech), but really deserve more accurate titles, and

Table 3.5 Types of apraxia and their localizations

Types of apraxia	Localization
1. Limb kinetic	Basal ganglia, supplementary motor area (SMA)
2. Ideomotor	Left parietal lobe
3. Ideational or conceptual	Left temporal lobe
4. Orobuccal (oral)	Left inferior lobe

will not be considered in this section. Four main types of motor apraxia are recognized (see Table 3.5).

Limb kinetic apraxia

Patients with this form of apraxia have a breakdown of fine motor organization and the co-ordination of finger movements necessary to perform fine motor tasks. They are particularly poor at copying meaningless hand positions and better when mimicking meaningful gestures (saluting, waving etc.) and typically use real objects flawlessly. This pattern is observed in patients with basal ganglia and supplementary motor area (SMA) pathology. It is characteristic and prominent in the early stages of corticobasal degeneration although other forms of apraxia are seen as the disease progresses.

Ideomotor apraxia

This disorder mainly accompanies aphasia but can be seen without a frank language disorder. Patients are unable to carry out motor acts to command, but typically perform the same acts spontaneously. There is difficulty with the selection, sequencing, spatial orientation, and movements involved in meaningless and meaningful gestures (waving, beckoning, etc.), and in demonstrating the use of imagined household items (for example, a toothbrush or comb) or tools. Imitation improves performance and patients are considerably better when using real objects.

In right-handed patients, ideomotor apraxia is associated with left hemisphere lesions. The critical areas are the inferior parietal and prefrontal areas. Such lesions may either destroy motor engrams (cortically stored movement patterns) or disconnect the flow of information necessary for initiating complex motor acts. Anterior callosal lesions can cause the inability of one limb—usually the left—to perform on command, even though the other limb performs normally.

Ideational or conceptual apraxia

The term **ideational apraxia** has been applied to the inability to carry out a complex sequence of co-ordinated movements, such as filling and lighting a pipe or making a cup of tea, although, in contrast to what happens in ideomotor apraxia, each separate component of the sequence can be successfully performed. This seems to be a very rare disorder and might relate more to frontal dysfunction. It has also been used to describe the inability to mime the use of objects (for example, a toothbrush) and, importantly, to use the actual object due to a loss of the underlying conceptual knowledge. Therefore a better term is **conceptual apraxia**. The issue of whether knowledge of object use constitutes a separable domain of semantic memory has been a topic of controversy. There are reports of patients with apparently isolated conceptual apraxia, although evidence from semantic dementia suggests a common integrated semantic system. This form of apraxia is seen in patients with semantic dementia and in advanced Alzheimer's disease. In the latter group it is difficult to unravel the contribution of apraxia from the confounding effects of poor language comprehension and diminished attention.

Orobuccal (oral) apraxia

Patients with oral apraxia have difficulty performing learned, skilled movements of their face, lips, tongue, cheeks, larynx and pharynx on command. For example, when they are asked to pretend to blow out a match, suck a straw, or blow a kiss, they make incorrect movements. The critical areas for lesions causing this deficit are the inferior frontal region and the insula. Thus oral apraxia commonly accompanies Broca's aphasia. Some of the speech-output deficits in Broca's aphasia may result from apraxia of speech (i.e. difficulty with articulation and phonation secondary to impaired motor programming). Orobuccal apraxia is also seen in patients with frontotemporal dementia, progressive non-fluent aphasia and corticobasal degeneration.

Damage to Specialized Right Hemisphere Functions

Deficits related to right hemisphere damage (in right-handed individuals) are much more difficult to detect than those caused by comparable dominant hemisphere damage. Often the deficits are subtle, and have not been noticed by the patient or observers (see Table 3.6). Thus it is arguably more important to assess any patient with suspected cognitive impairment carefully for these deficits, since aphasia and apraxia will usually be readily apparent.

It should also be noted that all of the functions described in this section are only **relatively lateralized** to the right hemisphere: spatial and visuo-perceptual skills are both bilaterally represented, but the hemisphere that is non-dominant

Table 3.6 Deficits arising from right hemisphere damage

1. Neglect phenomena*	
Personal:	Denial of hemiplegia (anosagnosia)
	Unconcern over deficit (anosodiaphoria)
	Neglect of grooming, shaving, etc.
Motor and sensory:	Hypokinesia
	Visual, auditory, and tactile neglect
	Sensory extinction to simultaneous bilateral stimulation
Extrapersonal:	Hemispatial neglect (e.g. drawings, line bisection, visual search)
	Neglect dyslexia and dysgraphia
2. Dressing apraxia*	
3. Constructional disorders*	
4. Complex visuo-spatial deficits*	Object recognition (apperceptive and associative agnosia, optic aphasia)
5. Deficits in face processing	Prosopagnosia
6. Disorders of colour perception	Achromotopsia, colour agnosia and anomia
7. Balint's syndrome	
8. Topographical disorientation	
9. Prosodic components to language, e.g. melody and intonation, especially emotional components (see p. 59–60)	
10. Vigilance/arousal, as part of attentional control (see Chapter 1)	

*NB: These functions are not very well lateralized, but deficits are more common and more severe with right hemisphere damage.

for language is more specialized with aspect to these abilities. The deficits described in this section are more severe and long-lasting with right hemisphere damage, but virtually all of them can be found to lesser degrees with left-sided lesions.

Neglect phenomena

There is substantial evidence that the right hemisphere in man is more important than the left for spatially directed attention. The term 'attention' is applied rather broadly in neuropsychology to a number of different phenomena. I have used the qualifier 'spatially directed' to separate this form of attention directed to personal and extrapersonal space from the more general meaning of attention in the context of concentration/attention, which was discussed in Chapter 1. Deficits in spatially directed attention produce unilateral neglect.

The term 'neglect' has been used to describe a complex of behavioural abnormalities. At its most profound, there is neglect of attention to both personal and extrapersonal space although these two phenomena are separable.

Personal neglect

In its most extreme form, patients behave as if one half—usually the left—of their body has ceased to exist. If hemiplegic, they deny any impairment, a phenomenon termed **anosagnosia**. They may even deny the existence of half their body, claiming that their left arm is someone else's. More frequently, patients admit that they have a neurological deficit, but appear unconcerned about it. This has been termed **anosodiaphoria**. Initially patients with neglect may ignore stimuli presented to the side contralateral to their lesion, whether the stimulus is visual, tactile, or auditory. Later, they become able to detect these stimuli, but when given simultaneous bilateral stimulation will fail to report the stimuli presented to the contralateral side. This phenomenon is called **extinction to double simultaneous stimulation**. It is most often observed in the visual and tactile modalities. Patients with severe personal neglect shave, groom and dress only their right side, and even eat the food on the right half of the plate only. Failure to move their head and eyes to the side opposite to the lesion and motor akinesia of the contralateral limb may also be observed.

Motor and sensory neglect

Motor or intentional neglect involves a response failure that cannot be explained by weakness, sensory loss or inattention. There may be failure to move a limb (**limb akinesia**) or the limb can be moved but only after a long delay and strong encouragement (**hypokinesia**). Patients with intentional neglect who can move may make movements of decreased amplitude. They may also have an inability to maintain postural movements, known as impersistence. Patients with motor neglect, who can move their contralesional limb, may fail to move this limb (or have a delay) when they are required to move their ipsilateral limb. Limb akinesia, hypokinesia, hypometria and motor impersistence can affect some or all parts of the body including the limbs, eyes or head. Patients with motor neglect may also have intentional biases such that there is a tendency to move towards the ipsilesional space.

The same type of phenomenon is seen in the sensory realm. Sensory neglect involves the selective defect of a deficit in awareness, which may apply to all stimuli on the affected side of space, or may be confined to stimuli impinging on the patient's body (personal neglect). The modalities affected by neglect may vary: subtypes of sensory neglect exist for the visual, auditory and tactile modalities. The deficit in awareness is accompanied by an abnormal attentional bias.

Once attention is engaged on the ipsilesional side, subjects may have difficulty disengaging their attention and moving to the contralateral side. If the lack of awareness and attentional bias are present only when there is a competing stimulus at the ispilesional location, the disorder is known as **extinction**. Many patients with sensory neglect recover and become able to detect isolated contralesional stimuli but continue to manifest extinction most typically in the visual or tactile realm.

Extrapersonal neglect

This is usually tested by asking patients to bisect lines of varying length, to perform cancellation tasks or to draw and copy pictures. When asked to copy a drawing of an object such as a clock or house, patients typically fail to draw the left side. On line bisection tasks they place the half-way mark to the right of the mid-point which is particularly apparent using long lines. Tests involving the cancellation of letters or stars among other stimuli distributed across a page are particularly sensitive methods of detecting neglect. When writing they may leave a wide margin on the left or occasionally omit the initial part of the word (**neglect dysgraphia**). On reading, there may be omission of the beginning of the line or even the initial letters of a word (**neglect dyslexia**).

In milder cases there is often no external manifestation of neglect, and only through specific testing by drawing and cancellation tests will the impairment be detected.

Applied anatomy and causes of neglect

Neglect is very common in the acute stages following damage to either the right or left cerebral hemisphere, but it is usually short-lived. Severe persistent unilateral neglect is found most often following damage to the right inferior parietal lobe (Brodmann areas 29 and 30) and, to a lesser extent, after right dorsolateral prefrontal cortex damage. Homologous areas in the monkey receive inputs from the higher-order sensory association cortex, the thalamic nuclei, and parts of the limbic system (especially the cingulate cortex). Outputs go primarily to the frontal eye fields, the striatum and the superior colliculus. Thus the inferior parietal lobule can be considered as a centre for integrating sensory experiences, motivational responses, and visual search mechanisms. Although apparently widely distributed, these diverse brain areas (parietal, prefrontal and cingulate cortices, thalamus, and reticular system) are all intimately linked by reciprocal connections. Lesions of any one of these disrupt the mechanisms of spatially directed attention, and may therefore produce neglect phenomena. Acute frontal lobe injury usually results in ipsilateral head and eye deviation, accompanied by visual and personal neglect phenomena. Lesions of the thalamus, the basal ganglia, or the cingulate gyrus may also cause unilateral neglect. Neglect is most commonly observed in the context of strokes but is also found in association with tumours and occasionally in patients with neurodegenerative diseases.

Mechanisms of neglect

Many patients with unilateral extrapersonal neglect have accompanying hemianopia, and it is tempting to attribute neglect to the visual loss. However, neglect may also be seen in patients with intact visual fields, and many patients with complete hemianopia are able to orientate and follow into their blind half-field, and furthermore do not show neglect phenomena on drawing or cancellation tasks.

Attentional model

One popular model proposed to explain the occurrence of neglect after right hemisphere lesions is as follows. Whereas the left hemisphere contains mechanisms which maintain attention to the contralateral (right) half of the sensory world, the right hemisphere contains the neural apparatus for attending to both sides of space. Thus lesions of the left hemisphere produce no substantial deficit, since the intact right hemisphere can take over the task of attending to the right side. Right hemisphere damage, on the other hand, will cause left unilateral neglect, since the intact hemisphere lacks the mechanisms for ipsilateral attention (see Figure 3.5). To explain the phenomena of personal neglect, it has been proposed that the parietal lobe contains representations of the body with these same asymmetries. An elaborated version of the attentional model proposes that spatial attention is composed of three elementary processes: engaging, disengaging and shifting. Patients with right parietal damage are thought to have selective deficits in disengaging attention from stimuli to the right, resulting in an inability to shift and engage stimuli to the left. Recent work has also emphasized the deficit in spatial working memory found in neglect subjects: on cancellation tasks they are unable to keep track of which targets have been visited before, leading them to repeatedly go over and over the same spatial location.

Representational model

In a famous experiment carried out in Milan, patients with neglect were asked to describe the cathedral square as if standing on the cathedral steps overlooking the square. They accurately described the features on the right side of the square, but omitted the details on the left. They were then asked to imagine that they were standing at the opposite end of the square, facing the cathedral.

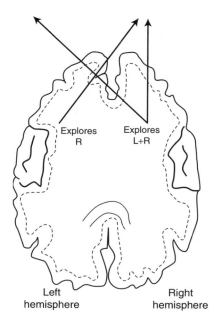

Explores
R

Explores
L+R

Left
hemisphere

Right
hemisphere

Fig. 3.5 A model of hemisphere specialization in directed attention in which only a right-sided lesion will lead to unilateral visual neglect.

Now, they described all the features to their right (which had previously been omitted) and neglected those to their left (which had previously been included). This neglect of internal imagery has subsequently been reported in many neglect patients, and can be tested at the bedside by asking patients to imagine that they are walking down a very familiar street and to describe all the buildings they would pass. Representational theories propose that the inability to form an adequate contralateral representation underlies the clinical phenomena of neglect. It is postulated that the right hemisphere is responsible for constructing a central map of space which is a direct analogue of sensory experience.

At present, there is no entirely satisfactory unitary hypothesis to explain the diverse phenomena observed in neglect patients. It is probable that both attentional and representational models are, in part, correct.

Tests for unilateral neglect (see Chapter 5 and the Appendix for details)

1. Generating representational drawings to command (for example of a bicycle, a house, etc.).

2. Copying of symmetrical drawings (for example of a two-headed daisy, a clock-face, etc.).

3. Line bisection, in which the subject has to mark the half-way point on a number of lines of variable length.

4. Letter or star cancellation—in these tests the subject is given a piece of paper covered with randomly distributed letters or stars or a mixture of both and is asked to cancel the target items (for example, the small stars).

5. The Behavioural Inattention Test is a standardized battery for detecting and measuring the severity of visuo-spatial neglect.

Dressing apraxia

A disturbance in the ability to dress is fairly common following focal right hemisphere damage and more diffuse brain injury. The term 'apraxia' is inappropriate, since it is not a motor disorder. Instead, the deficit is in the orientation of body parts in relation to garments because of faulty visuo-spatial mechanisms. When there is a focal lesion, it is usually in the right posterior parietal area. Other phenomena of right hemisphere damage are invariably present. Patients with more advanced dementia or acute confusional states (delirium) may show the same problem.

Constructional disorders

Impairment in the ability to copy a visually presented model by drawing or assembling blocks has been termed constructional apraxia. As with dressing apraxia, this bears little relation to motor disorders.

To copy adequately a two-dimensional shape, such as a cube or star, requires normal visual acuity, the ability to analyse and perceive the elements of a drawing, and, finally, co-ordinated visuo-motor ability. Given the complex nature of the task, it is not surprising that deficits can arise with right- or left-sided cerebral damage. However, constructional apraxia is more common, and more severe, in patients with lesions of the right hemisphere, especially if the parietal lobe is involved. There are also qualitative differences. Left-sided lesions lead to over-simplification in copying. Right-sided cases make gross alterations in the spatial arrangement, with so-called 'explosion' of the constituent parts. Constitutional deficits are seen in patients with Alzheimer's disease, particularly the visual variant, and are severe in patients with corticobasal degeneration.

Tests of constructional ability (see Chapter 5 and Appendix for details)

1. Copying three-dimensional shapes (for example, a cube) or the overlapping pentagons from the Mini-Mental State Examination and the clock-drawing test (see ACE-R, p. 157).

2. Copying the Rey–Osterrieth Complex Figure.

3. Block design from WAIS.

Complex visuo-perceptual abilities

Although both hemispheres are involved in the processes of visual analysis, there is evidence for right hemisphere specialization. Patients with right-sided lesions have more substantial deficits on a range of visuo-perceptual tasks, including:

1. 'Unusual views' tests, in which subjects are asked to match photographs of the same common objects photographed from conventional and from more unusual viewpoints, or to identify objects photographed from unusual viewpoints.

2. Tests in which subjects are asked to identify items in overlapping line-drawings, or from partially degraded or fragmented images.

3. Judgement of line orientation, which requires the subject to match a single test line to lines in a larger array.

4. Tasks requiring the analysis and matching of faces, often photographed from different angles and with different lighting conditions.

A battery of standardized tests for the detection of abnormalities of this type, the Visual Object and Space Perception Battery (VOSP, see Appendix is available, but is not suited to routine bedside use.

Subtle deficits in perceptual processing are impossible to detect at the bed-side; but severe disorders of visuo-perceptual processing may result in various forms of visual agnosia, which should be recognizable clinically.

Visual object agnosia

The term 'agnosia' can be roughly translated as 'non-recognition'. Visual agnosia implies a disorder of recognition that cannot be attributed to general intellectual impairment, aphasia, or basic sensory dysfunction. A patient with visual object agnosia sees objects, but fails to recognize what they are. Agnosias may be visual, tactile, or auditory. Within a particular modality, agnosia can occur for different classes of stimuli such as colours, objects, or faces. Often patients are agnosic for more than one class of items, and sometimes in more than one modality. Since visual object and face agnosia are most common, I have concentrated on these.

There are two principal types of object recognition disorder: one involves the earlier perceptual stage of object analysis; in the other there is a breakdown in the processes by which meaning is ascribed to visual percepts (see Figure 3.6).

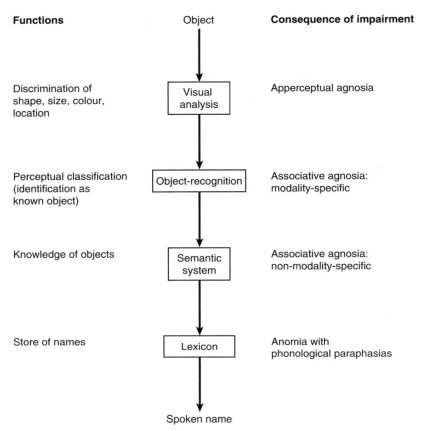

Fig. 3.6 A cognitive model of object recognition, understanding, and naming.

These disorders have been termed 'apperceptive' and 'associative agnosia', after the work of Lissauer in the late 19th century (see Table 3.7).

Apperceptive visual agnosia

Patients with this form of visual agnosia show preserved elementary visual faculties, such as acuity, simple shape and contour discrimination, and colour perception, but fail on more complex tasks involving object identification and naming. They are typically unable to copy shapes, or to discriminate two examples of the same object in arrays.

Visual fields may be normal; but most patients have defects on perimetry ranging from left hemianopia to marked tunnel vision. Despite being unable to identify visually presented objects, patients retain full knowledge about the unidentified items, and can name them by palpation or if given a verbal

Table 3.7 The differentiating features of apperceptive agnosia and associative agnosia

	Basic visual processing	High-level perceptual analysis	Naming and identification	Semantic knowledge
Apperceptive agnosia	✓	✗	✗	✓
Associative agnosia	✓	✓	✗	✗/✓

*In some cases semantic knowledge is preserved, whereas others show a pervasive disorder of object knowledge.

✗, impaired; ✓, preserved.

description. For instance, if shown a watch, patients with apperceptive agnosia would be unable to identify it as such, but if allowed to hold it would name it correctly. If asked to name the item 'worn on the wrist and used to tell the time' they would have no difficulty retrieving the word 'watch'. The lesion in apperceptive visual agnosia usually involves fairly widespread bilateral posterior occipitoparietal regions. Interestingly, carbon monoxide poisoning appears to have a particular aetiological role. Cases with bilateral posterior watershed strokes, penetrating head injury, and mercury poisoning have also been described.

Associative visual agnosia

This term has been applied rather loosely to patients with the inability to recognize visually presented objects despite apparently normal high-level perceptual processing. In classic cases the deficit is confined to the visual modality, while in others the deficit is more pervasive and multimodal (in more modern terminology the latter is referred to as a loss of semantic knowledge). The specific disorder of optic aphasia (see p. 88) is also sometimes included in this category.

Classic (modality-specific) associative agnosia This is extremely rare. Patients have difficulty identifying or naming visually presented objects. Preservation of high-level perceptual processing can be demonstrated by their normal drawings of objects they cannot recognize, and by their ability to match pairs of such stimuli as the same or different. The traditional interpretation of this deficit considers the functional lesion to be one of accessing stored semantic knowledge from the visual modality, as a result of a disconnection in the flow of information (see Figure 3.6). More recently it has been shown that high-level perceptual processes may not be entirely normal—patients are consistently better at recognizing real objects than photographs or line drawings, and the naming errors are invariably visual in nature. The site of pathology in such patients is variable: all have posterior quadrant damage, and in many it is bilateral; but cases with left unilateral posterior temporoparietal lesions have also been documented.

Cross-modal associative agnosia In most cases of associative agnosia there is a generalized semantic memory impairment. The defect in object recognition is, therefore, *not* limited to visual presentation. These patients demonstrate an inability to identify objects in any modality (for instance touch, or verbal description), as well as a loss of verbal knowledge which affects fine-grained (attributional) rather than broad category information. That is, they will be able to identify a picture as an animal, but unable to specify the type of animal. Likewise, on multiple-choice questions they will identify the word 'tiger' as the name of an animal, but make mistakes when asked about its size, habitat, ferocity, etc. A number of patients have been described in whom the loss of semantic knowledge is 'category specific', for instance affecting living but not man-made things, or vice versa. Such deficits are considered more fully in the section on semantic memory (see p. 19).

The locus of damage in patients with deficits in semantic memory invariably includes the left anterior temporal lobe. A degree of global semantic memory loss, resulting in features of associative agnosia, is present in patients with moderately advanced Alzheimer's disease, and to a more marked extent in patients with semantic dementia (see p. 45). Interestingly, in patients with 'category specific' loss of knowledge about living things the cause is very often *herpes simplex* virus encephalitis.

Optic aphasia

In this very rare syndrome, described by Freund in 1889, there is a disorder when naming or verbally describing visually presented items. In contrast to what is found in visual agnosia, patients with optic aphasia can recognize items visually, as demonstrated by their accurate pantomiming of their use, even though they cannot access their names. The deficit is modality-specific, in that naming by tactile presentation and naming to description (for example, what do you call 'a large triangular musical instrument with many strings played by plucking?') are intact. Various explanations have been advanced to explain this strange syndrome. One influential account postulates a disconnection between stores of visual and verbal semantic knowledge. Thus object presentation activates intact visual knowledge, but verbal semantics cannot be assessed via this route; whereas, when one is given a verbal description, there is no difficulty with name access. Most cases are associated with right-sided visual field defects, achromatopsia, and/or alexia, since the site of damage is usually the left medial occipital region.

Tests for the detection and classification of visual object agnosias (see Chapter 5 for details)

1. Object naming (patients with visual agnosia produce visually and semantically based errors) using pictures and real objects.

2. Object description and miming use.

3. Copying of drawings.

4. Naming to description (for example, what do you call the object 'worn on the wrist to tell the passage of time'?, etc.).

5. Ability to provide semantic information about unnamed items (for example, 'tell me everything you can about X').

6. Tactile naming.

The Cambridge semantic memory battery consists of a range of tasks based upon the same core set of 64 items (half natural and half man-made) with subtests designed to test input to and output from semantic knowledge about these items (see Appendix).

Prosopagnosia

This term describes the inability to recognize familiar faces. While patients state that all faces are unfamiliar or unrecognizable, they are able to use cues such as voice, gait, or distinctive clothing to identify familiar people.

Following contemporary models of cognitive processing, face identification proceeds from a perceptual to a recognition stage, whereby faces are categorized as familiar, and then compared with stored representations of known faces before the appropriate name can be produced (see Figure 3.7).

In prosopagnosia the deficit is at the categorization stage of this process, since these patients are able to describe and identify facial components (for example, beard, nose, etc.), match faces in arrays containing examples of the same and different faces and identify emotional expressions. In many cases they even retain the ability to perform complex visual matching tasks requiring the matching of faces taken under different lighting conditions and from different angles, although such tasks are usually performed slowly and laboriously. They also retain their knowledge of people they are unable to recognize, so that they may be unable to recognize a photograph of Margaret Thatcher, but when given the name can produce appropriate factual information. Not surprisingly, prosopagnosics are invariably impaired at learning new faces.

The question of how selective the deficit is to face processing is controversial; most, if not all, cases have problems with fine-grained identification such as types of flower, breeds of dog, makes of car, etc., leading some authorities to

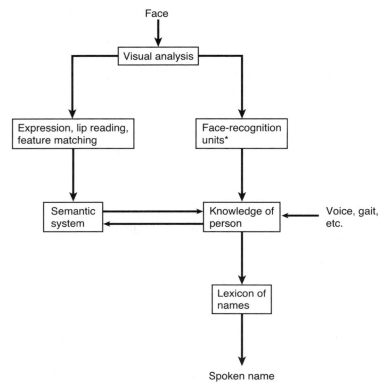

Fig. 3.7 A cognitive model of face recognition. Face-recognition units function as a memory store of known faces. A lesion at this level (*) causes prosopagnosia.

speculate that prosopagnosia is a defect in distinguishing items within categories containing many confusable exemplars.

Prosopagnosia is most commonly associated with bilateral inferior occipitotemporal lesions, but occasional cases with purely right-sided lesions have been reported. Field defects are usually present, and many patients have additional deficits such as achromatopsia or pure alexia.

A variant of prosopagnosia occurs in the context of anterior right temporal lobe atrophy which is a homologue of semantic dementia. Patients complain of progressive difficulty with face recognition and/or naming. Unlike post-stroke prosopagnosia the deficit is cross-modal. That is to say, they have difficulty identifying the people from their face *and* in producing information in response to the name (they are unable to name a photograph of Ronald Reagan, would not be able to name 'the President of the USA who was an ex-actor' and produce little, or no, information in response to the name). Another difference is that the deficit is dependent on the degree of familiarity: family, friends and extremely famous people are still recognized, at least in the early stages.

Tests of face processing (see Chapter 5 for details)

1. Naming and description of photographs of familiar famous persons

2. Matching of photographs in arrays containing examples of the same face (sometimes taken from different angles or in different lighting conditions) amongst other faces.

3. Identification of emotional expressions from faces.

Achromatopsia, Colour Agnosia, and Colour Anomia

Achromatopsia is an acquired disorder of colour perception characterized by a loss of ability to discriminate between colours. It may occur in isolation from other defects in object or form perception. It is usually symptomatic; patients complain that everything appears washed out, or 'like black-and-white TV'. It may affect part or the whole of the visual field. The critical site of pathology is the medial occipito-temporal region. Pure alexia (alexia without agraphia, see p. 70) and achromatopsia in the right hemifield often occur together after left posterior cerebral artery territory infarction.

In contrast, patients with **colour agnosia** are able to perceive and distinguish between colours, but are impaired on tasks requiring the retrieval of colour information (for example, 'What colour is a banana?'). A specific disorder in colour naming with preservation of colour perception and of colour knowledge has also been reported under the heading of **colour anomia**. The latter syndrome may also be associated with alexia and right hemianopia, and is attributed to a disconnection of the left hemisphere language centre from visual information.

Tests of colour processing

1. Colour discrimination (i.e. distinguishing colours and matching examples of the same colour in arrays).

2. Colour naming (i.e. producing the correct colour name when shown coloured objects or colour samples).

3. Colour knowledge (for example 'What colour is a banana?', etc.).

Balint's syndrome

This classic syndrome has three components: (i) psychic paralysis of gaze, that is to say an inability to direct voluntary eye movements to visual targets;

(ii) **optic ataxia**, the inability to reach for, or point to, visual targets, also referred to as visual disorientation; and (iii) a visual attentional deficit in which only one stimulus at a time is apparently perceived, and even the attended stimulus may spontaneously slip from attention; this last feature is termed 'simultanagnosia'.

Patients complain of severe visual difficulties, and may appear to be functionally blind. When faced with arrays of items or complex pictures they appear to be able to attend to only one small area at a time, with a resultant inability to synthesize the parts into a whole. Despite this severe limitation in what they can see at one time, visual fields may be full when they are challenged with gross stimuli. Patients exhibit a severe deficit in representing the relative location of objects relative to themselves, referred to as egocentric disorientation. More recent studies of patients with this pattern of deficits show consistent topographical disorientation, although this was not part of the original description. There are marked difficulties with spatial navigation.

The brain damage responsible is always bilateral, and includes the superior parieto-occipital region, damage to which interrupts the flow of spatial information from primary visual to parietal association areas. Cerebrovascular disease and prolonged hypotension leading to watershed infarction are the usual causes, although bilateral tumors and white matter disorders such as progressive multifocal leucoencephalopathy and mitochrondrial disorders may also result in the same syndrome. In an outpatient setting, the commonest cause is so-called **posterior cortical atrophy**, a variant of Alzheimer's disease (see p. 42).

Topographical disorientation

Considerable progress has been made in understanding the complex ability to navigate in previously familiar environments and to learn new routes quickly and without conscious effort. A loss of way-finding ability is known as **topographical disorientation** (see Table 3.8). The non-dominant parietal lobe, posterior cingulate, lingual and parahippocampal cortices all contribute and can be considered a topographical network.

There is a crucial distinction between, on the one hand knowing and learning the spatial relationship between objects and landmarks in the environment versus, on the other hand, problems in the recognition of familiar landmarks. As with amnesia, another important dimension is the difference between anterograde impairment (i.e. the ability to learn a new environment) versus problems recalling the spatial layout of previously known environments.

Lesions to the posterior parietal cortex (typically bilateral) cause great difficulty in representing the location of objects relative to self, known as egocentric disorientation. This is typically associated with components of Balint's syndrome

Table 3.8 Topographical disorientation

Egocentric disorientation	Inability to represent the location of objects relative to self Co-occurs with features of Balint's syndrome	Bilateral posterior parietal
Landmark agnosia	Inability to recognize salient environmental stimuli (buildings etc.) a form of associative agnosia	Lingual gyrus (basal occipital)
Anterograde spatial disorientation	Inability to create new maps or representations of the environment	Right parahippocampal gyrus (parahippocampal place area, PPA)

(see above) and is extremely disabling. A variant of this syndrome affecting the ability to judge the position from which photographs of familiar buildings or objects are taken has been described in association with right posterior cerebral artery infarcts.

The ability to acquire new internal maps of an environment depends upon the posterior parahippocampal gyrus, a region known as the parahippocampal place area (PPA). Patients with lesions to the right PPA are completely unable to learn new routes and appear unable to encode information about novel spatial relationships. In contrast to these problems with spatial relationships and spatial route learning, patients with basal temporal lesions involving the lingual gyrus may develop a form of agnosia analogous to prosopagnosia but involving the recognition of previously familiar buildings.

Chapter 4

Cognitive and Neuropsychiatric History Taking and Tips on Physical Examination

The Patient Interview

The importance of establishing an accurate and detailed account of the patient's cognitive problems and their evolution cannot be over-emphasized. It is also essential to obtain an independent account from the patient's spouse/partner or, if necessary, another family member or close friend. This applies particularly in the area of memory disorders and behavioural/personality change, where the patient is frequently unaware of his or her deficit. By the end of the interview it should be possible to formulate a fairly accurate provisional diagnosis, or at least to delineate the areas of cognitive function requiring particular attention on examination.

Suggested structure of interview

1. Introduce yourself and other staff present.
2. Outline the plan of the interview and examination.
3. Interview the patient, preferably alone, explaining that you wish to hear about his or her symptoms and problems. If the informant remains present, tell him or her that you would like to talk first to the patient without the 'help' of the relative. Make sure that you do talk to the patient alone at some stage; there may be important confidential facts that he or she wishes to impart, or personal questions that would be inappropriate with others present.
4. Interview the informant alone.
5. Physical and cognitive examination. Again, it is essential to do this with the patient alone to gain a true picture and to avoid embarrassing the patient and his or her family.

For the full assessment of a new patient we allow an hour, which is often not long enough for a full cognitive assessment, but this should allow a working diagnosis to be reached. Further neuropsychological testing will often be necessary.

Beginning

Before embarking upon the history of the presenting complaint, try to establish a rapport with the patient by asking a few general, non-confrontational questions about the patient's background, such as place of birth, schooling, past jobs, family, hobbies, and interests. Even at this stage valuable information is gained. Clearly, if the patient is unable to engage in sensible conversation and answer simple questions accurately and coherently, then further attempts to take a history from the patient in person will be impossible and pointless. In this situation the informant will be vital in providing information about the current problems and background.

Reason for referral

Does the patient know why he or she has been referred to the clinic, or why he or she is in hospital? In ordinary medical practice, we usually assume that patients are fully aware of the reasons for their referral. In patients suffering from cognitive deficit this is not always the case. It is revealing to enquire why they think they are being seen. Questions need to be phrased sensitively to avoid insulting or patronizing the patient, but can usually be achieved with something along these lines: "I like to ask all of my patients to tell me why they think they have been referred to see me." It is surprising how often patients think that they are being seen about a skin complaint or bad hearing!

Open-ended questioning

Continue the interview by asking general 'open-ended', rather than leading, questions. This provides the best opportunity to obtain a non-biased narrative account of the patients' problems. Some suggestions are:

+ Tell me how your problems first started.
+ What are your main areas of difficulty at present?
+ What impact has this had on your work, family, hobbies, etc.?
+ What are the activities that you are having difficulty with?

Try to record in the hospital notes phrases used by the patient verbatim. These are often much more meaningful and useful to future doctors than statements such as 'complaining of memory difficulties' or 'six years progressive dementia'.

Direct questions

In all cases the narrative account obtained by open-ended questions needs to be supplemented by questions designed to probe specific domains of cognitive function. In this way, an overall pattern of abilities in each area can be built up. Valuable additional information will be obtained by questioning the patient's relatives. Indeed, in more impaired patients this supplementary information is by far the most important. A check-list for use with patients and informants is given below.

Check-list for interviewing patients and informants

1. Memory	◆ attention and concentration
	◆ anterograde: recall of new episodic information in day-to-day life (for example, recalling messages and conversations, outings/trips, losing things, family news, TV programmes, etc.), repetitiveness, disorientation
	◆ retrograde: past personal and public event memory
	◆ semantic: vocabulary, memory for names and general factual knowledge (history, geography, etc.)
2. Language	◆ output: word finding, grammar, word errors (paraphasias)
	◆ comprehension of words and grammar
	◆ reading
	◆ writing: spelling and motor components
3. Numerical skills	◆ handling money, shopping, dealing with bills
4. Executive abilities	◆ planning, organization, problem solving, flexibility
	◆ hobbies, use of appliances
5. Visuo-spatial skills	◆ dressing
	◆ constructional abilities
6. Neglect phenomena	◆ bodily neglect
	◆ neglect of extrapersonal space
7. Visual perception	◆ recognition and identification of people
	◆ object and colour identification
8. Route finding and landmark identification	◆ recognition of known landmarks, ability to learn new routes
9. Personality and social conduct	◆ social conduct, empathy, egocentrism, disinhibition
	◆ sexual behaviour
	◆ eating, grooming, personal hygiene
10. Eating	◆ appetite, food preference, manners
11. Mood	◆ features of depression (including sleep, libido, appetite)
	◆ elation and mania
12. Motivation	◆ mental energy, get-up-and-go, drive

13. Anxiety or
    agitation
    ♦ irritability, restlessness, autonomic symptoms

14. Delusions
    ♦ delusions of theft, infidelity, phantom boarder,
      Capgras delusion

15. Hallucinations
    ♦ visual, auditory, tactile, olfactory

1. **Memory**

The complaint 'memory difficulty' is used in a variety of ways by patients and relatives. Try to establish if the patient is referring to one of the following three domains.

Attention and concentration

Symptoms of poor attention include the inability to concentrate when reading a magazine or book; difficulty following conversations although language comprehension is normal; immediate loss of new information, for instance following a telephone conversation; walking from one room to another and forgetting the reason why you wanted to go there; slips of everyday action such as putting the milk in the oven or the clean plate in the dishwasher etc.

These are all symptoms that we all experience at times of stress, when very tired or preoccupied. They are exaggerated in patients with depression and anxiety but are also the types of 'memory' symptoms that predominate in patients with frontal, subcortical and basal ganglia pathology.

Episodic memory

More commonly, in the context of a memory clinic, the symptom is applied to memory for personally experienced events or recently acquired information (messages, news items, shopping, conversations, etc.), in which case the deficit is one of episodic (event-based) memory.

An important distinction, clinically and neuropsychologically, is between memory for newly encountered information (anterograde memory) and memory for past events (retrograde memory). Usually these are affected in parallel, and to a roughly equivalent degree, for instance in Korsakoff's syndrome and Alzheimer's disease. However, dissociations may occur; after closed head injury there is severe anterograde amnesia and limited retrograde; with selective damage to the hippocampus fairly pure anterograde memory loss may occur.

In order to gain an overall impression of the severity of memory loss it is helpful to ask the patient to estimate the degree of impairment of day-to-day memory on a scale of zero (terrible, abysmal, no recall of new information) to 10 (fine for my age, as good as my friends). We ask this question of the patient and accompanying family member. Patients with organic memory loss typically give higher scores (e.g. 5 or 6) compared to their spouse (e.g. 2 or 3), whereas the opposite applies in patients with depression or anxiety, and the 'worried well'.

Confabulation refers to the tendency to produce erroneous material on being questioned about past events. Confabulations may occasionally be grandiose and delusional, but more commonly consist of mis-ordering and fusion of true past memories.

Semantic memory

Loss of memory for words and names or difficulty coming up with names is the principal symptom of patients with semantic memory impairment. Naming depends on both knowledge of the target and the linguistic components of name retrieval and articulation. It is important, therefore, to disentangle these aspects. Patients with semantic memory loss are fluent without phonological or syntactic errors in speech. When semantic memory breaks down it produces problems with word production and comprehension although the latter is much less evident to patients and their families. It is usually apparent when processing complex information, for instance when a number of people are talking or when trying to digest the meaning of written language containing less common words.

It is also important to enquire whether there has been a decline in the patients' general knowledge: most people have some fund of expert vocabulary related either to their work or hobbies.

Reminder: Throughout this book I avoid (wherever possible) the confusing terminology of short-term and long-term memory. In experimental psychology, short-term refers to the very limited capacity store, lasting only seconds as measured by digit span. Alternative names for this short-duration system are immediate or working memory. By contrast, clinicians and the general public usually refer to short-term memory as that assessed by name and address recall after 5 or 10 min (see p. 8 for a fuller discussion). Whenever I use 'short-term' it is in the neuropsychological sense.

Suggested areas of enquiry

Attention/concentration: Is the patient able to follow the plot in a book or film? Are there slips of everyday action, or poor concentration?

Anterograde episodic memory: Ability to remember new information, such as news stories, and important personal material, such as family events. Does the patient need to use lists more than in the past? Has he or she become repetitive? Does he or she frequently lose things while at home?

Retrograde memory: Recall of past personal events such as holidays, operations, jobs, and past homes. Recall of public and news items.

Semantic: Names of people, places, and things. Vocabulary and factual knowledge. Deterioration in this domain usually manifests as difficulty with naming and understanding the meaning of less common words.

2. Language

When questioning patients and their relatives about language problems it is useful to consider language in terms of production and comprehension.

Language production

+ Is the patient as fluent and articulate as normal?

+ Has there been a deterioration in grammar?

+ Is there a misuse of words (paraphasias)? Most patients with aphasia produce incorrect or distorted words in spontaneous speech. The occurrence of semantic (for example, SISTER for BROTHER, APPLE for ORANGE) and phonemic (SITTER for SISTER) paraphasias may be noted by relatives.

+ Is word-finding difficulty apparent? A degree of anomia, especially for less common words, is more or less a universal accompaniment of aphasia, and is frequent from the early stages in dementia of Alzheimer type.

Language comprehension

Disorders of language comprehension may affect grammar (syntax) or word meaning (semantics). It is difficult to tell these apart as both are often first apparent when trying to follow complex instructions and keeping track of group conversations. Using the telephone is particularly difficult for patients with any degree of comprehension deficit, because all the usual gestural and contextual cues to meaning are absent. Comprehension deficits parallel output disorders in that patients with non-fluent aphasia have difficulty understanding sentences while those with fluent anomic aphasia tend to have problems with word comprehension.

Reading

Can the patient still read fluently with comprehension and pleasure? A reduction in leisure reading is a subtle indicator of mild dyslexia; but memory and attentional difficulties may complicate interpretation of this symptom. In dominant hemisphere injury, reading problems usually accompany and mirror spoken language; but in occasional cases pure alexia may occur. The rare, but well-recognized, combination of alexia with preserved writing ability is a distinct and localizing syndrome, almost invariably associated with right hemianopia, and often with disorders of colour perception and verbal memory problems.

Writing

If a history of writing difficulty is elicited, try to distinguish between break-downs in spelling or in the motoric control of writing. In the latter, termed 'apraxic agraphia' which may occur in basal ganglia disorders, oral spelling is preserved. Remember, most people write very little other than shopping-lists and postcards. Agraphia is, therefore, usually underestimated by relatives and patients but is common in neurodegenerative diseases.

Note: disorders of reading and writing do not always denote dominant hemisphere pathology. In neglect dyslexia patients may fail to read one side—usually the left side—of the page or individual words. Likewise, in neglect dysgraphia one portion of the page or word is omitted. Consider these syndromes if other aspects of spoken language are normal.

3. Numerical skills

Difficulty with manipulating numbers often manifests as inability to use money, and hence to shop alone. Ask also about management of household accounts.

4. Executive abilities

As discussed in Chapter 1, this term refers to the uniquely human ability to initiate, plan and organize, which in turn involves goal setting and attainment while avoiding distractions and remaining flexible and responsive to changing contingencies. There is, of course, huge variability in baseline abilities in this domain so it is important to assess change from the patient's normal state.

Two types of questions are helpful. First, general enquiries about ability to plan, organize and solve problems plus signs of distractibility or impersistence. The second, and generally more informative, line of enquiry concerns executive function in action. That is to say, the patient's ability to organize his or her usual life: work, home commitments, use of appliances, DIY, hobbies, planning holidays and trips.

This is a domain where the family members' view is virtually always more informative. Patients typically lack insight into these problems which are all too evident to family, friends and colleagues.

5. Visuo-spatial skills

In contrast to language and memory disorders, which are usually clearly apparent to close observers, deficits in visuo-spatial ability may be clinically silent.

Therefore it is particularly important to make specific enquiries about potential symptomatology.

Dressing ability

Impairment in the ability to dress oneself, so-called dressing apraxia, usually reflects a complex visuo-spatial deficit rather than a true apraxic (i.e. motor-based) problem. The act of putting on a shirt requires alignment of body parts and mental rotation, which depend upon the non-dominant hemisphere. Thus this type of dressing disorder usually occurs in the context of focal right posterior parietal lesions. Patients with frontal brain damage may show a different disorder of dressing, which consists of a mis-sequencing of garments, and results in wearing underpants on top of trousers, etc.

Constructional deficits

These are rarely evident without formal testing. Occasionally patients with particular skills or professions (architects, model builders, etc.) may complain of difficulty drawing or in three-dimensional constructions, suggesting right parietal damage. It is always worth asking about hobbies. A specific decline in practical abilities such as DIY or drawing may also suggest right-sided pathology but often reflects impaired executive function.

Spatial orientation

Topographical disorientation, that is to say, getting lost in familiar surroundings, is a common accompaniment of moderately advanced dementia. It may also indicate focal right hemisphere pathology. It may be due to poor spatial memory or to failure to recognize landmarks.

6. **Neglect phenomena**

Neglect of space

Patients with focal right hemisphere lesions often fail to respond to stimuli in the opposite half of extrapersonal space. This may manifest as a failure to talk to visitors on the left side of the bed, a tendency to ignore food on the left half of the plate, constantly bumping into objects and door-jambs on the neglected side, or even failing to read the left half of the page.

Bodily neglect

In its most profound form, patients deny the presence of hemiplegia despite evidence to the contrary. The term 'anosagnosia' applies to this phenomenon. Less dramatic versions, consisting of a tendency to ignore or under-use one side, are more frequent.

7. Visual perception

Misidentification

Patients with disorders of visual processing may think that faces on the television are actually in the room. Misidentification of familiar faces may also occur, and is common in delirium, when other illusions and hallucinatory experiences are often present (see agnosia below).

Agnosia

There are a number of fairly rare syndromes involving the inability to identify faces, colours or objects despite normal basic perceptual processes. In prosopagnosia, patients are unable to recognize faces belonging to friends, acquaintances or famous people. They can, however, identify these people correctly from voice, dress, or gait. A failure to recognize people by any sensory modality suggests a deficit of semantic memory. In visual object agnosia, subjects fail to recognize objects by sight, but can still identify the same objects by touch. Achromatopsia denotes a loss of colour vision with preserved acuity and object identification. Suggestions for useful screening questions are:

- Does he or she ever confuse you or other family members with someone else?
- Have you noticed any problems in recognizing familiar faces?
- Has he or she had difficulty in identifying everyday objects, or used things inappropriately?
- Have you noticed any problems with colour vision?

8. Route finding and landmark identification

As discussed in Chapter 3, the ability to navigate in a complex environment depends on a number of cognitive processes, notably the recognition of familiar landmarks and learning and retaining spatial maps. Patients with posterior parietal and mesial occipital pathology are prone to topographical disorientation. This is very prominent in posterior cortical atrophy and in dementia with Lewy bodies.

9. Personality and social conduct

It is difficult to overlook major deficits in memory and language, even with unstructured history taking, and visuo-spatial disorders should be readily detected by a few simple pen-and-paper tests. Disorders of social cognition and conduct as associated with frontal lobe damage or disease, by contrast, are easily overlooked, and it is in these domains that informant interview is extremely important. One should ask if there have been any changes in character, personality or social behaviour.

Typical personality changes associated with frontal lobe dysfunction consist of lack of concern about oneself and others, often with childish, egocentric behaviour, inability to empathize, and lack of inhibition, with a tendency to react impulsively. A lack of spontaneity, with reduced initiation of conversation and activity is common. Patients have difficulty reading 'social' situations and the emotional state of others, leading to *faux pas* or gaffes. Not infrequently patients are aggressive toward family members. Relatives may note a deterioration in eating, grooming and toileting habits. A tendency to bawdiness, such as telling 'dirty' jokes or making inappropriate advances may be reported.

With bilateral temporal lobe damage, patients may develop features of the Kluver–Bucy syndrome, consisting of a tendency to eat indiscriminately, sometimes including inedible items (cigarette-ends, soap, etc.), without satiety, altered sexual drive, emotional blunting and passivity.

10. Eating, appetite and food preference

Changes in eating behaviours are common in psychiatric illness and in fronto temporal dementia. Reduced appetite and weight loss are important biological signs of depression. Increased appetite with a craving for sweet foods, often coupled with rather stereotyped patterns, such as insisting on exactly the same meal every day for dinner, is typical of frontotemporal dementia. Patients may also suddenly decide to become vegetarian or alternatively switch after many years to eating meat. Many of those with more advanced Alzheimer's disease suffer reduced appetite but food fads and cravings are unusual.

A decline in table manners is also a feature of frontal type dementias. Any hint of dysphasia should ring alarm bells for the presence of motor neuron disease but it also occurs in basal ganglia disorders, especially progressive supranuclear palsy.

11. Mood

Atypical depressive illness is undoubtedly the commonest treatable disorder in patients presenting to a memory disorder clinic. Complaints of poor memory's and especially of an attentional type, which are in excess of those noted by others, should make the clinician consider an affective illness. Besides obvious questions about spirits and mood, the following are useful lines of enquiry:

1. Lack of pleasure from life (anhedonia).

2. Preoccupation with pessimistic thoughts about the past and future; feelings of worthlessness.

3. Inappropriate guilt.

4. Loss of interest in work, the family, home, and hobbies.

5. Recurrent thoughts of death and suicide.

6. Poor concentration.

7. Reduced energy and fatigue.

8. Biological features, especially disturbances of sleep with early morning wakening and a diurnal variation of mood, loss of appetite and libido, elevated mood with a pervasive feeling of well being (elation) coupled with hyperactivity and racing thoughts suggest hypomania.

12. Motivation

You should always enquire about interest level or 'get-up-and-go' since apathy is a very common feature in organic brain disease and in depression. Apathy consists of a lack of motivation and diminished goal-directed behaviour with decreased emotional engagement. Although it is a common accompaniment of depression, it is often an independent manifestation of brain disease and has been attributed to anterior cingulate dysfunction. It is typically accompanied by dysexecutive features.

13. Anxiety and agitation

Anxiety is characterized by agitation and unjustified apprehension, feelings of forebodings and thoughts of impending doom. Patients are irritable, tense and have poor concentration. Autonomic disturbances (sweating, palpitations, nausea, dry mouth and lightheadedness) are common. Restlessness, pacing and fidgeting should also alert you to significant anxiety. Anxiety is a common early feature in all forms of dementia.

14. Delusions

Delusions are false beliefs based on incorrect inferences about external reality that are firmly held despite evidence to the contrary. Delusions in dementia typically focus on theft of property, burglary, and infidelity. In the **Capgras delusion** the sufferer claims that people are not who they claim to be or have been replaced by an imposter. There may be delusions of reduplication, i.e. thinking that there are multiple versions of a spouse or of a place. In the phantom boarder delusion patients believe that other (often unwelcome) people are living in the house. Any of these delusions may occur in demented patients but appear more common in dementia with Lewy bodies. In idiopathic psychotic disorders, such as schizophrenia, delusions are commonly accompanied by evidence of thought disorder. Bizarre and religious delusions are rare in dementia. Grandiose delusions suggest mania.

15. Hallucinations

Hallucinations are sensory perceptions that have the same compelling sense of reality as true sensory experiences but occur without stimulation of the relevant sensory organ. In neurological patients, visual and olfactory hallucinations are commoner than those in the auditory modality. Fairly often there is also at least partial insight. A particular form of visual hallucination, which involves seeing well-formed, and often remarkably realistic, images of animals, faces, and often children, is common in patients with dementia with Lewy bodies and in more advanced Parkinson's disease, when it is usually secondary to dopaminergic medication. It has been termed peduncular hallucinosis, since it was originally described in association with acute vascular lesions of the cerebral peduncles in the mid-brain. Formed visual hallucinations in the absence of cognitive impairment are known as the **Charles Bonnet syndrome.** Most patients with this disorder have poor eyesight. Vivid hallucinations are common in acute confusional states, when tactile hallucinations of crawling or itching may also occur. Olfactory and gustatory hallucinations are invariably fleeting, and may occur as part of the phenomena of complex partial seizures originating from the medial temporal lobe. Hallucinations may be mood-congruent in patients with depressive or manic psychosis.

A sensitive way of enquiring about such phenomena is to say something like the following: "Patients with various kinds of neurological disorder sometimes have unusual experiences when they see, hear, or smell things which may not be there. Have you had anything like that?"

When talking to relatives you should ask specifically whether the patient has ever seemed to be seeing or hearing things, or talking to non-existent people.

The Informant Interview

The general format of the informant interview should follow that used with the patient. General open-ended questions should be used first, followed by directed questions to cover each area of cognitive function. Establishing the evolution, pattern, and impact of the deficits is the overall aim.

What were the first observed problems?

In the dementias this is particularly important, because in their end-stages all degenerative diseases tend to produce an indistinguishable picture. The earliest-noted deficit is thus of important diagnostic value. For instance, if there is an insidious decline in anterograde memory, with preservation of personality and social behaviour, then the diagnosis is almost certainly Alzheimer's disease. Early change in personality and social conduct points to frontotemporal dementia.

Word-finding difficulty or speech hesitancy localizes the process to the dominant hemisphere. Spatial disorientation or dressing apraxia as the predominant problem alerts the clinician to the right hemisphere, and so on.

Was the onset acute, insidious, or stuttering?

The mode of onset of cognitive problems is very important. Delirium is always abrupt in onset, and often fluctuating in its course. If an apparent dementing syndrome has an acute or subacute onset over days or weeks, then a depressive pseudodementia should be suspected. The rate of progression is also helpful diagnostically: Alzheimer's disease progresses insidiously, multi-infarct dementia typically has a step-wise course, dementia with Lewy bodies is associated with fluctuations and Creutzfeldt-Jakob disease progresses extremely rapidly.

Situation-based problems

Instead of sticking to questions purely about individual cognitive domains it is often illuminating to enquire about particular difficulties in various everyday settings, such as:

- at work
- cooking and general housework
- driving
- using money and paying bills
- gardening and other hobbies
- social encounters with family and friends

Impact on the family and personal relationships

Assessment of the impact of any cognitive change on the family is clearly very important. This also gives the opportunity to enquire about sexual activity. Contrary to the views of the young, sexual intercourse does not stop at forty, or even necessarily at seventy. Most spouses dealing with difficult and embarrassing changes in sexual behaviour will value your interest in this sensitive area.

Family History

It is inadequate to record in the medical notes 'Family History: nil relevant'. This is best exemplified by apparently *de novo* cases of Huntington's disease in which a family history is frequently said to be 'negative'. Detailed probing about the family background invariably reveals important clues, such as an uncle who committed suicide or a grandfather who died at a young age in a mental hospital.

Besides noting the age, state of health, and cause of death of first-degree relatives, preferably in the form of a family tree, you should ask specifically about any family history of neurological or psychiatric illness. As most patients have no idea what constitutes illness in these areas, ask specifically about:

+ senile dementia
+ memory loss
+ Alzheimer's disease
+ Parkinson's disease
+ epilepsy
+ strokes
+ mental breakdowns
+ depression
+ suicide

Also enquire whether any family members have ever needed to see a psychiatrist.

Past Medical History

Of particular importance in assessing cognitively impaired patients are the following:

1. Significant head injury, i.e. injury associated with post-traumatic amnesia of more than one hour, neurosurgical procedures, skull fracture, or post-traumatic seizures.
2. Epilepsy of any type.
3. Previous CNS infections, either meningitis or encephalitis.
4. Psychiatric illness.

Alcohol Intake

Opinions as to a reasonable level of alcohol intake vary considerably. Women are undoubtedly more susceptible to alcohol-mediated complications than men. The working party of the Royal College of Physicians recommend 'safe levels' of up to 21 units/week for men and 14 units/week for women. The same report suggests that 'hazardous' levels are 21–49 units/week for men and 14–35 units/week for women. 'Dangerous' levels are above these limits. Try to record the average weekly intake in numbers of units per week. One unit is equivalent to half a pint of beer, one small glass of wine, or a measure of spirits. People often underestimate the extent of their alcohol intake, and it is often very useful to go through the last week on a day-to-day basis, adding up everything they recall drinking. An independent assessment of alcohol intake should always be sought from the patient's spouse.

Tips on Physical Examination

It is not appropriate to describe here the complete neurological examination which should obviously be performed on all patients presenting with cognitive disorders. I shall concentrate instead on a few additional, and perhaps less commonly known, signs which are useful in the detection of focal cerebral abnormalities.

Cranial nerve signs

Smell

I do not test smell routinely. It should, however, be tested in the following circumstances: past history of head injury; dementia, especially of frontal lobe type; complaints of poor taste or smell; and the presence of visual symptoms or signs (suggesting subfrontal pathology).

Vision

As well as testing acuity (in each eye) and pupillary responses and fields, remember to examine for visual extinction or neglect in every patient. Visual extinction is the consistent tendency to ignore stimuli in one half field (or, rarely, one quadrant) when both sides are simultaneously stimulated by finger wiggling. The visual fields must first be shown to be intact when using single stimuli. Visual extinction is always pathological, and implies damage to the opposite posterior parieto-occipital area. Although included in the category of neglect phenomena it occurs commonly with right- and left-sided brain damage. This is a good time to test for optic ataxia (visual disorientation) by asking the patient to touch your fingers whilst wiggling them in each quadrant with the patient fixating ahead. Whilst looking at the eyes also remember to observe for Kayser–Fleisher rings. These brown pigmented rings or crescents are best seen with the patient looking down whilst illuminated with a torch from the side, and are pathognomonic of Wilson's disease.

Eye movements

Abnormalities are most often missed because of hasty examination and a failure to test vertical eye movements. Gaze should be sustained in each of the primary positions, i.e. horizontal right and left, vertical up and down. As well as following (pursuit) movements, testing should include rapid voluntary side-to-side and vertical (saccadic) movements. These may be selectively disrupted in basal ganglia disorders (for example Huntington's disease). A severe and selective deficit in vertical eye movements occurs in progressive supranuclear palsy (Steele–Richardson–Olzewski syndrome) (see p. 50), and also following upper brain-stem and thalamic strokes.

Frontal release signs

A large number of primitive frontal signs have been described. These reflexes are released from normal inhibition in the presence of frontal lobe damage or disease. Their interpetation is difficult, because some occur in a high proportion of the normal elderly, and they rapidly fatigue on testing. In descending order of usefulness they consist of:

1. *Grasping*. This is practically always pathological below the age of 80 years. To elicit, lightly stroke your hand across the patient's palm whilst distracting the patient with casual conversation. A positive response consists of involuntary grasping, which can be fairly subtle. The patient does not have to grasp your hand like a vice for it to be abnormal!

2. *Pouting*. Ask the patient to close his or her eyes lightly. Place a spatula in the mid-point of his or her lips in the vertical plane. Warn the patient that you will tap the spatula firmly, but not too hard. A positive response consists of puckering of the lips towards the stick, as if to blow a kiss. This may be normal above the age of 70 years.

3. *Glabellar tap*. With the patient sitting, tap gently and repetitively with the index finger in the mid-line between the eyebrows, keeping the rest of your hand out of view. Normal subjects blink in response to the first two or three taps only. Continued blinking after five or more taps is considered positive. Many of the normal elderly have a positive glabellar tap.

4. *Palmo-mental response*. This is the least meaningful of the frontal release signs. It is elicited by stroking the thenar eminence with an orange stick or a similar implement, and observing the contralateral mental muscle, which is situated on the chin. A positive response consists of the contraction of this muscle.

Motor system

Postural arm drift

This is tested by asking the patient to maintain a static position of the outstretched arms in the horizontal position with the eyes closed. Downwards and usually inwards drift of the arm is a frequent sign of contralateral hemisphere disease, and may be found in the absence of any other motor signs. Observation of the hands and fingers in this position is also very useful for detecting involuntary choreiform or dystonic movements.

Involuntary movements

These are best observed when taking the history. Chorea is often overlooked, and attributed to fidgetiness. If there is any doubt about their presence, ask the patient to lie still on the bed with the eyes gently closed. Also watch when the patient is walking; this often exacerbates chorea, producing characteristic finger-flicking movements, and may also bring out dystonic limb-posturing.

Sensory system

Astereognosis

This is a form of tactile agnosia in which the patient is unable to recognize objects despite normal sensation, co-ordination and motor function. Deficits are associated with contralateral parietal lesions. It occurs equally with right- and left-sided damage.

Graphathesia

The inability to recognize letters or numbers traced on finger tips is also associated with damage to the somatosensory parietal cortex. A few practice numbers should be drawn for the patient with the eyes open, making sure that the numbers traced out are oriented towards the patient.

Sensory inattention

This denotes a failure to appreciate a stimulus when a similar stimulus is applied simultaneously on the opposite side. For instance, patients can register when their right hands are touched, but when both sides are simultaneously touched they report only the left-sided stimulation. This method is often called double simultaneous stimulation. It occurs frequently with right and left parietal lesions.

Gait and balance

No neurological examination is complete without watching the patient rise from a seated position and walk twenty paces or so. Impairment in the initial stages, with the 'glued to the floor' sign, is characteristic of gait apraxia associated with normal-pressure hydrocephalus. Small-rapid festination, with a hunched posture and lack of arm swing, characterizes Parkinson's disease. Particular difficulty with turning or changing direction is a common accompaniment of Parkinson's disease and other degenerative extrapyramidal disorders (such as progressive supranuclear palsy). The choreiform movements of Huntington's disease are frequently exacerbated by walking. Visual neglect may be apparent if the patient consistently bumps into objects to one side. When sitting, patients with progressive supranuclear palsy tend to collapse backwards *en bloc* rather than adjusting their back and leg positions as normal.

The 'stork' manoeuvre

If the patient can balance on one leg with arms folded across his or her chest and with eyes open, then any significant disorder of balance and practically any lower limb pyramidal weakness can be excluded.

Chapter 5

Testing Cognitive Function at the Bedside

The general schema followed is that already outlined in Chapters 1 and 3. The first part of the examination should assess distributed cognitive functions; deficits in these indicate damage to particular brain systems, but *not* to focal areas of one hemisphere. The second part of the assessment should deal with more localized functions, divided into those associated with the dominant (i.e. the left side, in right-handers) and non-dominant hemispheres.

The Addenbrooke's Cognitive Examination (ACE), which has now been revised (ACE-R), is described in Chapter 7. The ACE-R takes approximately 15 min to complete and can be regarded as a basic screening instrument that is particularly useful in an outpatient setting. It was developed principally to aid in the detection and monitoring of dementia syndromes and is less valuable in the diagnosis of delirium or other cognitive disorders. Specific shortcomings and pitfalls are discussed below, and in the context of the illustrative cases in Chapter 8.

Cognitive assessment should always follow history taking, because invaluable information is gained from the patient and informant, which guides the examination. For instance, even minor degrees of aphasia should be apparent from history taking, and will lead the examiner to assess language function thoroughly.

General Observations

Mood and motivation are essential to all mental functions. The degree of co-operation, the ability to sustain effort, and the amount of encouragement required to complete a task are all observable aspects of motivation. A disturbance in motivation is described as 'apathy', and if it is extreme the term 'abulia' is used.

Behaviour during the examination should be noted. Does the patient interact appropriately? Frontally damaged patients are often inappropriately jocular, or make puerile or obscene comments. Patients with acute confusional states (delirium) show either increased or decreased psychomotor activity. In the former state, patients are restless, voluble, noisy, fidgety, and distractable. In the latter, hypo-alert variant of delirium, patients are quiet, speak little, and drift easily off to sleep if unstimulated.

Orientation and Attention

The examination should begin by testing the patient's orientation and attention abilities (see Table 5.1).

Alertness

Record the level of wakefulness of the patient. It is hopeless to attempt a detailed cognitive assessment in a drowsy patient. A common-sense description such as 'awake and fully co-operative', 'co-operative but sleepy, with a tendency to doze off if unstimulated', are much better than vague, undefined terms such as 'obtunded' or 'stuporose'.

Orientation

This is conventionally divided into time and place. Of these, the first is the most important and clinically helpful.

Table 5.1 Summary of bedside testing for orientation and attention

Alertness	Level of wakefulness and reactivity	
Orientation	◆ Time	Day of week Date Month Season Year
	◆ Place	Building Floor Town County Country
Attention/concentration	◆ Serial subtraction of 7s ◆ Months of year backwards ◆ Days of week backwards ◆ Digit span forwards and backwards ◆ Formal tests: Stroop Test, Speeded letter cancellation tasks, Trails A, and the Test of Everyday Attention (TEA) which consists of a number of subtests designed to assess subcomponents of attention. The PASAT test and components of the CANTAB battery (see Appendix)	

Time

Time orientation should always include the day of the week, date, month, season, and the year. Date orientation is the least reliable, since some normal subjects do not know the exact date. When assessing inpatients the question 'How long have you been in hospital?' is often helpful. Even mildly delirious patients frequently over- or underestimate the passage of time, thinking that they have been in hospital for days when, in fact, they were admitted only that morning.

Disorientation in time is common in patients with acute confusional states (delirium) due to metabolic disorders or diffuse brain injury. It is also seen in patients with moderate-to-severe (but not mild) dementia, due to a combination of amnesia and attentional deficits, and in the amnesic syndrome.

Note: many patients with clinically significant memory impairment remain well orientated in time. Orientation in time should not, therefore, be taken to exclude a significant memory disorder.

Place

I usually use a question along the lines of, 'What is the name of this building?' It is surprising how often patients are unaware that they are in hospital, a fact that is easily overlooked if the examiner simply asks for the name of the hospital. Orientation in place is less sensitive than time orientation to attentional and memory deficits. The Mini-Mental State Examination (MMSE) and the ACE-R include orientation for town, county and country but these can usually be omitted in bright, alert and other well-oriented patients.

It is rare for patients to be unable to tell you their names. Even very confused or demented subjects do not show this deficit. But it is a characteristic feature of psychogenic (hysterical) amnesia. Aphasic patients may also be unable to access their own names, but when given a choice, such as 'Is your name Frank, John, or Harry?', can usually pick out the correct name. Patients with aphasia are frequently misdiagnosed as confused because they are unable either to comprehend the question or to produce the correct answer. This error should be avoided if the patient is engaged in casual conversation before plunging into formal cognitive assessment. Also included as part of person orientation are age and date of birth.

Attention/concentration

Ability to sustain attention and keep track of ongoing events can be assessed in a number of ways, including digit span, serial subtraction of 7s, spelling of familiar words backwards (for instance WORLD—DLROW), and recitation of the days of the week or the months of the year in reverse order. The two alternatives in the MMSE (serial 7s and WORLD backwards) are problematic.

Many normal elderly subjects make errors of serial subtraction, as do patients with focal left hemisphere damage and the scoring of omissions, substitutions and reversals is complicated. In the MMSE and ACE-R subjects are asked to spell WORLD backwards if they make any errors on the serial subtraction task. The scoring system is explained on p. 168. Recitation of the months of the year are an overlearnt sequence, familiar to everyone. The ability to recite these in reverse order is therefore a good measure of sustained attention. Patients should be fast and errorless at this simple test. If the patient is unable to do this, try the days of the week backwards instead.

Digit span

Digit span, especially reverse digit span, is a more accurate measure of attentional processes, and a useful adjunct to the measures above. The ability to repeat a string of digits has little, if anything, to do with the processes involved in laying down and retrieving new episodic (event) memories. Digit repetition depends upon short-term (working) memory, which in turn depends upon frontal executive and phonological processes (see p. 8). Reduction in digit span is a feature of impaired attention, as found in acute confusional states or moderate-to-severe dementia, and may also occur in patients with focal left hemisphere lesions. Patients with aphasia typically have a reduced digit span.

Note: patients with the amnesic syndrome (for example, Korsakoff's disease or early Alzheimer's disease), who may be totally unable to lay down any new episodic memories, have a normal digit span.

Digit span is tested by asking the patient to repeat a progressively lengthening string of digits. It is usual to start with three digits. Two trials are given at any level. If subjects pass on the first or on the second trial, then the next-length sequence is administered. Digit span is the highest level at which the patient passes *either* trial (see Box 5.1). The number should be read by the examiner at a rate of one per second—without clustering, which aids repetition: you only have to think of the usual way in which we recall telephone numbers.

Box 5.1 Forward digit span: example

6–2–7 correct
8–3–6 not administered
1–7–4–9 incorrect
7–2–5–1 correct
4–9–3–1–6 incorrect
3–8–4–7–9 incorrect
Forward span = 4 (impaired)

Exactly the same technique is employed on reverse digit span; however, here the patient is required to repeat the numbers in reverse order. It may be necessary to give some patients several demonstrations at two digits. Normal digit span is 6 ± 1, depending upon age and general intellectual abilities. Thus an intelligent young adult would be expected to have a forward span of at least 6. In the elderly, or those of low intellectual ability, 5 can be considered normal. Reverse span is usually one less than forward span (see p. 8 for further details). Digit span was not included in the ACE-R since it is quite time consuming and prone to produce erroneous results if numbers are clustered.

Episodic Memory

As has been previously discussed in greater detail (see chapter 1), there are many subcomponents to memory. To recap: in psychology, short-term memory applies to the system of working memory responsible for the immediate recall of small amounts of verbal or spatial information (tested at the bedside by digit span or immediate recall of a name and address), which bears little relationship to other aspects of clinically important memory. What we normally think of as memory—the capacity to learn and recall personally experienced events such as a meeting yesterday or last year's holiday—comes under the heading of episodic memory.

In clinical terms, episodic memory function is best considered as anterograde (i.e. the ability to learn new information) and retrograde (i.e. the recall of old information) (see Table 5.2). This distinction is particularly useful since different pathological processes may differentially affect one or other of these components. Semantic memory describes our permanent store of knowledge about things in the world, as well as about words and their meanings.

Anterograde verbal memory

An informal, but often very revealing, impression of memory can be gained by asking patients to recall the details of very recent events, such as their journey to hospital, what they watched on TV last weekend, or events on the ward. As a naturalistic test of episodic memory, I frequently employ the following technique: at the beginning of the interview, in the course of our general conversation, I find a topic of interest, such as the patient's family or a recent holiday, and tell the patient something about my own interests, family or holiday. Then later I ask the patient to recall these facts.

Name and address recall

As part of the ACE-R we ask the patient to repeat a simple seven-part name and address. This is repeated three times, even if entirely correct on the first or second

Table 5.2 Episodic memory function

Anterograde verbal	◆ Incidental recall of earlier conversation, journey to hospital, events on ward, etc.
	◆ Recall of three items from MMSE
	◆ Name and address learning, recall and recognition in ACE-R
	◆ Formal tests: story recall (logical memory); word-list learning tests (Rey Auditory Verbal Learning Test; California Verbal Learning Test, etc.); parts of the Doors and People Test; paired associate learning and other components of the Weschler Memory Scale
Anterograde non-verbal	◆ Recall of shapes
	◆ Formal tests: Rey–Osterrieth Complex Figure Test; Recognition Memory Test (faces); Pattern–spatial associative paired learning test or PAL from the CANTAB computerized battery
Retrograde	◆ Famous events, for example: Recent sporting events (world cup, olympics etc.) Political events, elections etc. Royal family news Wars and coups (Iraq, Afghanistan, Gulf, Falklands) Scandals (Blunkett affair, Monica Lewinsky affair, Watergate) Disasters (Tsunami, 9/11 Twin Towers attack, Herald of Free Enterprise, Brighton hotel bombing, Hillsborough stadium)
	◆ Remote personal (autobiographical) memory: Autobiographical Memory Interview (AMI)

trial, to ensure that it has been attended to and processed. Since repetition is within the span of short-term (working) memory, this is a measure of general attentional processes rather than of memory proper. After approximately 10 min (the actual time is not critical), after completing the rest of the ACE-R, the patient is asked to recall the name and address. It should be noted that this is a relatively crude measure. Total failure, or recall of one or two elements, is clearly abnormal at any age. Completely correct recall shows that the patient does not have a *major* amnesic deficit, although some patients shown to have a significant memory deficit on formal testing score perfectly on this simple task. Intermediate results are always more difficult to interpret. The revised ACE-R contains a recognition component which is administered for those elements that patients have failed to recall. Patients with true amnesia typically fail on the recall and recognition components or improve only slightly when given a choice, 'was it Kingsbridge, Dartington or Exeter?', whereas patients with anxiety, depression and frontal retrieval-based memory problems typically improve markedly. Thus the discrepancy between recall and recognition can be clinically very helpful. Clinical intuition is important. If informants are concerned about a patient's memory, even if the defect is not obvious on simple testing, then formal neuropsychological evaluation is required.

Formal assessment

For those interested, and who do not have access to professional neuropsychological assessment, I would recommend two measures: story recall (logical memory) and word-list learning. Both are quick and relatively foolproof. Furthermore, there are good normative data to guide interpretation. Several versions of stories for recall exist, all of which derive originally from the Wechsler Memory Scale. There are numerous word-list learning tasks. One of the most widely used is the 15-item Rey Auditory Verbal Learning Test (RAVLT) which consists of five learning trials, of list A, then an 'interfering' list B followed by recall of A again, and finally, after 20 min, a delayed recall of list A and a yes–no recognition phase. Another commonly used test in Memory Clinics is the Grober–Buschke Selective Reminding Test. Examples of these tests are given in the Appendix. For a more thorough evaluation of memory abilities, the Weschler Memory Scale—III, the Rivermead Behavioural Memory Test (RBMT) or the Doors and People Test are excellent all-round memory assessment instruments.

Anterograde non-verbal memory

In the vast majority of patients with memory disorders, non-verbal memory parallels verbal memory. Damage to the non-dominant—usually right—medial temporal lobe structures may, however, cause a selective non-verbal memory problem, such as a difficulty with learning faces, geometrical figures, or routes. Patients with early Alzheimer's disease are also typically impaired on tests of non-verbal memory such as the Paired Associate Learning (PAL) test from the computerized CANTAB battery. Unfortunately there is no easily administered bedside test of non-verbal memory. Spatial learning can be tested by walking a route around the ward or clinic with the patient, and then asking him or her to repeat this route alone. *Ad hoc* tests of face memory can be made using photographs from magazines of non-famous faces. The Rey–Osterrieth Complex Figure Test provides very good information on non-verbal memory. The subject is first asked to copy the figure (which is obviously a test of visuo-spatial skills), and then, after a delay of 30–45 min, without being forewarned, the subject is asked to reproduce the figure from memory. Normative data are available.

The Recognition Memory Test is a valuable standardized test of verbal and non-verbal recognition memory. In the face memory subtest, subjects are shown 50 faces, each for 3 s, and asked to make a value judgement as to whether they find the face pleasant or not. After finishing this part of the test, they are then given 50 pairs of faces, each containing one of the previously encountered faces, and asked to say which they have seen before. Normals perform surprisingly well on this test, and good normative data are available. The Rivermead Behavioural Memory Test also contains subtests that assess picture (object) recognition and recall of a route around the room (see Appendix).

Retrograde memory

Assessment of retrograde or remote memory is impressionistic at best, but a reasonable overall picture can be achieved by systematic questioning about a range of past events from the preceding months, years, and decades. Interpretation must be tempered by the patient's probable baseline performance. For instance, elderly women are unlikely to know in detail about recent sporting events, and many normal subjects' grasp of political events is extremely sketchy! Recall is harder than recognition, so start with open questions, such as 'Can you tell me about any recent news items?' or, 'What important events have been in the news lately?' Amnesic patients often have a rough idea, so it is important to probe for specific details. It is useful to ask about a standard list of famous events, examples of which are given in Table 5.2. In many patients with retrograde memory impairment, there is a temporal gradient. That is to say, they are much better at more distant events, and become progressively more impaired the nearer you get to the present. Patients with diencephalic amnesia (for example Korsakoff's syndrome) and Alzheimer's disease have a very extensive remote memory impairment. In pure hippocampal damage the retrograde loss may be more limited—a year or two at most although this is a controversial topic (see p. 15).

The other domain of remote memory is personal or autobiographical memory. An impression of the patient's capacity in this area is best formed during history taking. Can the patient accurately relate, and in the correct chronological sequence, events and details of his or her own life? The best formal test of remote personal memory is the Autobiographical Memory Interview (see Appendix).

Semantic Memory

Since semantic memory underlies so many aspects of cognition—our ability to produce and understand words, interpret pictures and recognize faces etc.—there is no single test of semantic memory. Deficits are typically detected using verbal tasks but are also present when patients are tested using non-verbally based tasks (see Table 5.3).

Category fluency is a very sensitive task but is also affected by other factors such as executive function. The interpretation of verbal fluency tests is discussed below (see p. 24).

Table 5.3 Tests for semantic memory functions (See Appendix)

- Category fluency (generation of exemplars from categories such as animals, fruit, etc.)
- Naming pictures
- Tests of verbal knowledge (generation of definitions from words or pictures)
- Picture pointing in response to the spoken name
- Non-verbal tests such as the Pyramids and Palm Trees Test or the Camel and Cactus Test from the Cambridge Semantic Memory Battery
- Person knowledge tests

Confrontation naming also detects semantic deficits with the production of broad subordinate responses (e.g. ANIMAL for RHINOCEROS, or MUSICAL THING for HARP). To confirm that the anomia is not due to a perceptual deficit, or simply due to word-finding problems, it is important to check that visual processing is intact and to probe knowledge in other ways. The former can be done easily by asking the patient to describe the unnamed pictures or to copy the drawings. Patients with semantic dementia can typically identify that something is an animal but have no idea about what kind of animal it is. They can also copy the line drawings and match together two drawings of the same thing. The fact that their problem reflects breakdown in underlying semantic knowledge is confirmed by word definition tests. If unable to name a picture of a rhinoceros, they typically can produce only very limited information in response to the name 'rhinoceros'.

The ability to point to a correct target in response to the command 'point to the rhinoceros' is critically affected by the foils. That is to say it is much easier if all the other possible choices are non-animals and hardest if they are other foreign animals. Tests using non-verbal materials such as the Pyramids and Palm Trees Test of associative knowledge are required to confirm the presence of a semantic memory deficit but these are beyond the realm of bedside testing.

Most patients with semantic deficits are particularly poor at naming and identifying famous faces but those with right temporal lobe damage show selective and often profound difficulties in this domain.

Frontal Executive Functions

The history obtained from an informant and general clinical observation of the patient's behaviour are more important than formal bedside testing for the overall assessment of the higher-order or executive functions. However, there are a number of measures which can be helpful in confirming clinical impressions (see Table 5.4).

Table 5.4 Tests for the assessment of frontal executive functions (see Appendix)

Initiation	◆ Verbal fluency tests: Letter fluency (F, A, S) Category fluency (Animals, Fruit, Vegetables)
Abstraction	◆ Proverb interpretation, e.g. 'A rolling stone gathers no moss' 'Too many cooks spoil the broth' 'Still waters run deep' 'A bird in the hand is worth two in the bush' ◆ Similarities test, e.g. 'apple and banana' 'coat and dress' 'poem and statue' 'table and chair' 'praise and punishment' ◆ Formal test: Cognitive Estimates Test (see Appendix)
Problem solving and decision making	◆ Formal tests: Tower of London Test (see D-KEFS test) or the Stocking of Cambridge version in the CANTAB battery and The Iowa or Cambridge Gambling Test from the CANTAB battery
Response inhibition and set shifting	◆ Alternating sequences ◆ Go-No-Go Test ◆ Motor sequencing tests (Luria Three-step and alternating hand movements) ◆ Formal tests: Wisconsin Card Sorting Test (WCST) and Trail Making Test: Part B (see Appendix). The CANTAB battery includes a test similar to the WCST, the ID-ED shift test, as well as other tests of working memory and mental flexibility. The Stroop Test. The Behavioural Assessment of the Dysexecutive Syndrome (BADS) consists of more ecologically based tasks such as the six elements, zoo map and key search subtests. The Hayling and Brixton tests are also useful recent tests of response inhibition and anticipation.

Initiation: verbal fluency tests

The generation of words beginning with a specified letter, or from a common semantic category (for example animals, fruit, etc.) depends on the co-ordinated activity of two main cerebral areas—the frontal lobes (which generate retrieval strategies) and the temporal lobes (where semantic knowledge is stored). Therefore, in the absence of a semantic deficit or aphasia, verbal fluency is a good test of frontal lobe function. In the standard version of the letter fluency test, patients are asked to generate as many words as possible, excluding names of people or places, in 1 min. The most commonly used letters are F, A and S. Normal young subjects should produce at least 15 words for each letter. A total for FAS of less than 30 words is abnormal; but some allowance should be made for age and background intellect. In the ACE-R we use the letter 'P' and calculate a scaled score of 0–7 depending on the number of novel correct words produced (see p. 169)

In category fluency tasks, subjects are asked to generate as many examplars as possible from semantic categories such as animals, fruit, vegetables, etc. For the category animals (used in the ACE-R), normal subjects produce around 20 items in a minute; 15 is a low average, and 10 is definitely impaired. Performance drops with age, and for the very elderly 10 may be just about acceptable. A reversal of the usual pattern (animals better than letter 'P') is highly suggestive of a semantic memory deficit.

As well as absolute numbers on both tasks, a note should be made of the number of perseverative responses. Normals do not perseverate. Patients with severe amnesia may produce perseverative errors; but in general they are a feature of frontal lobe disease or dysfunction of frontal lobe connections (for example, Huntington's and Parkinson's diseases).

A related and clinically useful task is the Supermarket Fluency Test: subjects are asked to list all the things that can be bought in a supermarket. Normal subjects systematically search various subcategories (dairy produce, fresh fruit, etc.), giving a few examples of each. On this test around 20 items is average, 15 is poor and below 10 is definitely impaired. Patients with frontal dysfunction show poor organization strategies and perseverative responses. In Alzheimer's disease, the patients attempt to search various categories, but produce few exemplars.

Abstraction: proverbs, similarities, and cognitive estimates

Some impression of abstract conceptualization can be gained from proverb interpretation and the similarities test. Suggestions of proverbs for adminis-tration are given in Table 5.4. Concrete interpretation, with an inability to make analogies, characterizes the performance of patients with frontal lobe damage: for instance 'too many cooks spoil the broth' is typically interpreted by such patients as referring to the cooking and making soup rather than its more general or abstract meaning. Interpretation of proverbs is highly dependent upon educational level and cultural background. Concrete responses may also be given by patients with schizophrenia.

The similarities test involves asking subjects in what way two conceptually linked items are alike, starting with simple pairs such as 'apple and banana' and 'table and chair', and progressing to more abstract pairs such as 'poem and statue' and 'praise and punishment'. The normal response is to form an abstract category (for example fruit, furniture, works of art). Patients with frontal deficits and dementia make very concrete interpretations (for example, table and chair:

'you sit at one to eat from the other' or 'both have legs') and often continue to do so despite being asked to think of other ways in which the items are alike.

Another useful test of conceptualization is the Cognitive Estimates Test, in which patients are asked a range of questions that require common-sense judgement to answer. Examples are 'How fast do horses gallop?', 'What is the height of the London BT Tower?', 'What is the height of an average Englishwoman?' and 'How many camels are there in Holland?'. Frontal patients give bizarre and illogical answers to these questions. The full test is given in the Appendix.

Response inhibition and set shifting

The ability to shift from one cognitive set to another, and to inhibit inappropriate responses, cannot be easily tested at the bedside.

Wisconsin Card Sorting Test

The best formal test of set shifting is the Wisconsin Card Sorting Test (WCST), which also involves problem solving and hypothesis testing. The subject has to sort cards containing geometric forms which differ in number, shape and colour. Having deduced the correct sorting dimension, the subject is then required to shift to another dimension (for example, from colour to shape) on a number of occasions. Patients with frontal lesions are unable to shift from one sorting criterion to another, and make perseverative errors. The Appendix contains a fuller description.

Alternating Sequences Test

This test is insensitive except in patients with gross deficits. The examiner produces a short sequence of alternating square and triangular shapes (see Figure 5.1). The patient is asked to copy the sequence, and then to continue the same pattern until the end of the page. Patients with frontal lobe deficits may repeat one of the shapes rather than continuing to alternate the pair.

Go-No-Go Test

Response inhibition can be tested using this paradigm. The patient is asked to place a hand on the table and to raise one finger in response to a single tap, while holding still in response to two taps. The examiner taps on the undersurface of

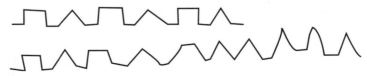

Fig. 5.1 An example of a frontal patient's copy of an alternating sequence.

the table to avoid giving visual cues. Patients with frontal deficits cannot inhibit raising one finger in response to the 'no-go' signal. Again, this is a relatively insensitive test, so that any abnormality is highly pathological.

Trail Making Test

This is a good quantitative measure of mental speed, attention shifting and response inhibition. On Part A, the patient must draw a line connecting randomly arranged numbers in numerical sequence (1–2–3, and so on). On Part B, the numbers are intermixed with letters, and the test is to draw a line connecting numbers and letters in an alternating sequence so that the connecting line goes from 1 to A to 2 to B to 3, and so on. Performance is influenced by intelligence and age. Age norms are available. An example of the test and normative data are given in the Appendix.

Motor Sequencing: The Luria Three-step Test and the Alternating Hand Movements Test

Deficits in sequencing complex motor movements are associated particularly with left frontal lesions. A number of tasks can be used, of which the 'Luria Three-step' and Alternating Hand Movements Tests are most helpful. In the former, the examiner demonstrates the series of hand movements—fist, edge, palm—five times without verbal clues, and then asks the subject to repeat the sequence (see Figure 5.2). Patients with frontal deficits are unable to reproduce the movements, even if given specific verbal clues.

In the Alternating Hand Movements Test the examiner again demonstrates the movement. The examiner starts with arms outstretched, one hand with fingers extended and the other with clenched fist. Then the hand positions are reversed by alternately opening and closing each hand in a rhythmical sequence (see Figure 5.3).

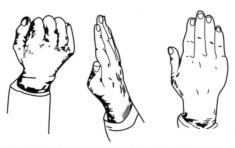

Fig. 5.2 Luria Three-step Test: the sequence of hand positions (fist–edge–palm) is shown. Figure taken from *Higher Cortical Functions in Man* by A. R. Luria. © 1966, 1979 by Aleksandr Romanovich Luria. Reproduced by permission of Basic Books, a member of Perseus Books Group.

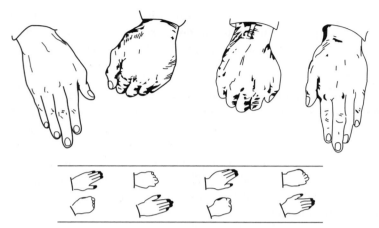

Fig. 5.3 Alternating Hand Movements Test: the hand positions (above) and the sequence of movements to demonstrate to the patient (below) are shown. Figure taken from *Higher Cortical Functions in Man* by A. R. Luria. © 1966, 1979 by Aleksandr Romanovich Luria. Reproduced by permission of Basic Books, a member of Perseus Books Group.

Dominant (LEFT) Hemisphere Functions

The second part of the bedside cognitive assessment should address more localized functions associated with the dominant and non-dominant hemispheres. Functions associated with the left hemisphere, which is dominant for right-handers, are language, calculation and praxis. Bedside assessments include the following.

1. Language
    A. Spontaneous speech during conversation and picture description:
       - Articulation
       - Fluency
       - Syntactic (grammatical) form
       - Paraphasic errors
       - Word-finding
       - Melodic line (prosody)
    B. Naming:
       - Overall ability
       - Error types
       - Benefit from cueing with initial sound

    C. Comprehension:
- Conversational understanding
- Pointing to command:
  Single-word (semantic)
  Sentence (syntactic)

    D. Repetition:
- Words and sentences

    E. Reading aloud and comprehension; if defective analyse the following:
- Letter identification
- Type of errors
- Effects of regularity
- Non-word reading

    F. Writing:
- Spontaneous writing
- Writing to dictation
- Oral spelling (if deficit is found in written spelling)

2. Calculation
- Number reading and writing
- Arithmetic operations

3. Praxis
- Buccofacial
- Limb gestures to command and imitation
- Object use

Language

Spontaneous speech

The analysis of spontaneous speech is a vital aspect of language assessment for the classification of aphasia. This should be done after listening to several minutes of spontaneous conversation and after asking the patient to describe a complex scene such as the one shown on p. 180. However, it should be noted that this analysis is much more readily applied to aphasia resulting from strokes and other focal lesions than to the aphasia seen in patients with degenerative brain disease. Deficits can be considered under the following headings.

1. *Articulation*: are the words well-formed and articulated, or laborious and distorted? Disturbances of phonetic aspects of language often accompany anteriorly placed or deep left hemisphere lesions.

2. *Fluency*: does the patient produce normal-length phrases between pauses? This should be disentangled from word-finding difficulty. Many patients with otherwise fluent aphasia have word-finding problems that break up their speech, but they are capable of producing occasional long phrases (five or more words). Patients with non-fluent speech have a consistently low rate of production in terms of words per minute, and produce short phrases. Phrase length should, therefore, be judged only after listening to several minutes of speech.

3. *Syntactic (grammatical) form*: does the patient produce speech that obeys the rules of his or her native language? Agrammatic speech is simplified, lacks grammatical words (pronouns, prepositions, etc.) and contains errors of tense. Agrammatism correlates closely with non-fluent language.

4. *Paraphasic errors*: are word-substitution errors present? These may be sound-based (phonemic paraphasias) such as SITTER for SISTER, or FEN for PEN. Or they may be meaning-based (semantic paraphasias), as are JUG for GLASS and APPLE for ORANGE. Severely paraphasic speech may contain non-words (neologisms), and in its most profound form produces jargon aphasia. Neologisms also occur in schizophrenic speech, but there they tend to be bizarre words used consistently, rather than with variable phonetic blends that characterize aphasia.

5. *Word-finding*: does the patient's speech have pauses followed by circumlocutions (for instance, 'the thing you write on paper with') or clichés such as 'thingy' or 'whatsit'?

6. *Melodic line (prosody)*: does the patient's speech have a normal intonation and stress, with a pattern of rising and falling pitch? Disturbances in prosody often accompany poor articulation and reduced fluency. Patients with laboured and awkward speech output are unable to maintain a melodic contour. Disturbances of emotional prosody (i.e. of inflection, tone and pitch used to express emotional states) may occur in right hemisphere damage.

Naming

The ability to name objects or pictures is impaired in virtually all aphasic patients, and is probably the best index of overall severity. A range of items of varying similarity should be used, since aphasics, in common with normal subjects, show a marked frequency effect. That is to say, they are much more likely to show errors when naming low frequency (less familiar) objects. This can be assessed using everyday items and parts of objects. Watch and pen are high-frequency items; winder, buckle and nib are low-frequency items. The type of error which occurs is also helpful diagnostically. Patients with anterior

(Broca's type) aphasia typically produce the initial sound of a word, and are helped by phonemic cueing. Conduction aphasias produce multiple phonemic errors (TELOP, TELE, TELEPHONT for TELEPHONE). Semantic paraphasias (for example CLOCK for WATCH, APPLE for ORANGE) are frequent in Wernicke's aphasia, sufferers from which may produce totally neologistic utterances. Semantic errors also characterize the anomia of Alzheimer's disease. Patients with semantic dementia are typically very anomic and produce semantic errors and particularly broad subordinate responses ('animal', 'musical thing' etc.). It should be remembered that accurate identification of visually presented objects also depends upon intact perceptual processes; the occurrence of visually-based naming errors and difficulty in visual identification in the absence of other language deficits should suggest a visual agnosia (see p. 85). There are several easily administered formal tests of naming ability, including the Graded Naming Test and the Boston Naming Test (see Appendix). The ACE-R includes 12 line drawings: two easy items (watch and pencil) from the MMSE and 10 harder items (five animals and five objects).

Comprehension

It is common to overestimate the comprehension abilities of aphasic patients on the basis of their understanding of unstructured conversation. In free conversation there are gestural, facial and prosodic (tone-of-voice) cues. Thus, fluent aphasics can often respond appropriately to opening conversational gambits ('How are you today?'), despite profound comprehension problems. Body-part commands may also be very misleading; responses to axial commands such as 'Close your eyes', 'Open your mouth', and 'Stand up' are commonly preserved. The reason for this preservation is obscure.

However, testing comprehension with difficult three-part commands (for example, 'Touch your left ear with your right index finger and then touch my hand') leads to erroneous *underestimation* of the comprehensional abilities, since these commands are not only grammatically complex, but also overload short-term (working) memory capacity, and require right–left understanding.

Comprehension is best tested by asking the patient to point first in response to single words and then in response to sentences of increasing complexity.

1. *Single-word comprehension*: It is possible to test understanding of words using everyday objects carried in your pocket (for example, a coin, a pen, a watch, keys, etc.) and items in the ward or clinic (for example, a bed, a chair, a desk, flowers, etc). Ask the patient to point to each in turn. Remember to use a spectrum of items of differing familiarity and parts of objects, since comprehension is always affected by this variable; severe aphasics may be able to point to the common but not the less common ones.

The ACE-R includes four questions involving the line drawings used for naming: "point to the one with a nautical connection" (anchor), "the one associated with the monarchy" (crown), "the one found in the Antarctic" (penguin) and "the marsupial" (kangaroo).

2. *Sentence (syntactic) comprehension—'The Pen–Watch–Keys Test'*: Again this can be easily performed using an array of three common objects from your pocket. Having established that the patient can understand the name of these items, test comprehension using a range of syntactic structures, such as:

'Put the pen on the watch.'

'Touch the watch with the pen.'

'Touch the keys and then the pen.'

'Touch the pen before touching the keys.'

'Touch the pen but not the keys.'

'Put the pen between the watch and the keys.'

'You pick up the watch and give me the pen.'

The most widely-used formal test of language comprehension is the Token Test, in which the subject has to follow commands of increasing syntactic complexity. The Test for the Reception of Grammar (TROG) was developed to assess language development but is very useful in assessing adults with suspected syntactic disorders (see Appendix). The most frequently used aphasic test, the Boston Diagnostic Aphasia Examination, includes tests of word and sentence comprehension as does the Western Aphasia Battery developed in London, Ontario.

Repetition

Repetition should be tested with a series of words and sentences of increasing complexity. It is best to start with short single words, and then to progress to polysyllabic words and finally sentences. The sentences should include ones that are rich in small grammatical function-words, which are particularly difficult for aphasic patients. Patients can then be graded on their ability to repeat accurately. The contrast between repetition and comprehension is often very informative in separating patients with semantic dementia from those with progressive non-fluent aphasia (PNFA). The former have no difficulty repeating words such as "hippopotamus" "eccentricity" "unintelligible" and "statistician" (the words in the ACR-R) but have no idea of their meaning. By contrast, those with PNFA show the opposite profile: impaired repetition but good understanding. Phrases without meaning such as 'no ifs, ands, or buts' are usually more difficult than sentences like 'The orchestra played and the audience applauded.'

Aphasics who cannot repeat have lesions involving the peri-sylvian language structures. Disproportionately severe breakdown of repetition is found in conduction aphasia and in patients with so-called speech apraxia who make gross phonetic errors with omissions, substitutions and distortions when repeating. Lesions outside the primary language zone and progressive degenerative disorders spare repetition, producing what are termed transcortical aphasic syndromes (see p. 58).

Reading

Both reading aloud and reading comprehension are important, but must be carefully distinguished. Failure to comprehend is usually accompanied by incorrect reading aloud. However, there are patients who cannot read aloud correctly, but have good understanding. If the patient successfully reads words and sentences, the capacity to read and understand a short paragraph should be tested. Simple reading comprehension can be tested by writing down a command such as 'Close your eyes' or 'Place your hands on top of your head if you're aged over sixty.' More complex comprehension can be assessed by asking the patient to read a paragraph from the newspaper and then asking questions about the content.

In most instances reading skills parallel spoken language abilities. But occasionally alexia may occur with agraphia, but without other aphasic deficits. Even more rarely, alexia may exist without even agraphia; this is called 'pure alexia' or 'alexia without agraphia'.

Once a reading problem has been uncovered, the next step is to determine which aspects of the normal reading process have broken down. The various types of dyslexia have been described (see p. 69), and consist of:

1. Pure alexia: letter-by-letter reading.
2. Neglect dyslexia.
3. Central (linguistic) dyslexias: surface, deep, etc.

Letter identification Errors in single-letter reading and the strategy of laboriously naming each letter (letter-by-letter reading), sometimes aided by tracing the letter outline with the finger, are characteristic of pure alexia.

Types of reading errors Reading a word as another conceptually related, but not sound-related, word (ACT for PLAY, SISTER for UNCLE, OCCASION for EVENT) is seen in deep dyslexia in which visual errors are also common (SHOCK for STOCK, CROWD for CROWN, etc.). Errors confined to the initial part of the word occur in neglect dyslexia (for example, FISH for DISH) secondary to right hemisphere damage.

Effects of word regularity Selective difficulty reading words that do not obey the normal sound-to-print rules of English—so-called 'exception words'—with a tendency to produce regularization errors (PINT to rhyme with MINT) is the defining characteristic of surface dyslexia. In the context of progressive neu-rodegenerative disorders the finding of surface dyslexia points strongly to a diagnosis of semantic dementia.

Non-word reading Patients with deep dyslexia, in which there is a breakdown in the sound-based reading route, are unable to read plausible non-words (NEG, GLEM, HINTH, DEAK, etc.). In deep dyslexia other deficits are present; but in phonological dyslexia the only major problem is with reading these nonsense words.

To screen for dyslexic syndromes, the list given in Table 5.5 contains non-words, regular words and exception words of mixed frequency. The ACE-R contains an abbreviated list of six exception (irregular) words.

Writing

Writing ability can be analysed in terms of the manual execution of writing, recall of individual letters and words, and sentence composition. Three major types of dysgraphia are recognized (see p. 73):

1. Dyspraxic dysgraphia.
2. Neglect or spatial dysgraphia: line- and word-based neglect.
3. Central (linguistic) dysgraphias: surface (lexical), phonological, and deep.

The type of writing disorder can usually be determined by spontaneous writing, writing to dictation, and oral spelling.

Spontaneous writing It is usually sufficient to screen for dysgraphia by ask-ing patients to compose a sentence about a subject of their choice. If they are unable to think of anything, suggest a recent journey or a description of their home. Defects in letter formation, spelling, and grammatical composition

Table 5.5 A word-list for screening dyslexic syndromes

Exception words		Regular words		Non-words
Pint	Soot	Shed	Board	Neg
Gauge	Steak	Nerve	Bridge	Glem
Sew	Suite	Wipe	Gaze	Gorth
Naïve	Aunt	Ranch	Flame	Mive
Thyme	Tomb	Swerve	Mug	Rint
Mauve	Height	Hoarse	Vale	Plat
Epitome	Dough	Sparse	Pleat	Hinth
Cellist	Sieve	Scribe	Ledge	Deak

should be readily apparent. If errors occur, then analysis of the specific deficit is required.

Note: it is not adequate merely to sample a patient's signature. Many severely dysgraphic patients maintain the ability to write their name, which can be thought of almost as an automatic reflex activity.

Writing to dictation To analyse the type of linguistic deficit in writing it is useful to have a list that contains words with regular sound-to-spelling correspondence and words with exceptional spelling. The list suggested above for reading will also serve this purpose.

Oral spelling If the disorder of writing appears to be motoric, in that individual letters are poorly formed, reversed, or illegible, then it is useful to check oral spelling, which is normal in dyspraxic and neglect agraphias.

Calculation

We do not routinely assess numerical and calculation abilities in our memory disorders clinic unless there is a suggestion of deficits in this domain on patient and/or carer enquiry or the patient is aphasic.

Number reading and writing

Number reading and writing should be assessed before arithmetic abilities by asking the patient to do the following:

1. Read a series of simple (7, 2, 9, etc.) and complex (27, 93, 107, 1226, etc.) numbers written by the examiner.
2. Write numbers to dictation.
3. If there are errors then it is helpful to examine the patient's ability to copy and point to numbers on command.

Arithmetic operations

Only after number reading/writing has been assessed should the patient's ability to understand arithmetic operations be assessed as follows:

1. Calculation skills should be tested by asking the patient to perform oral arithmetic calculations that sample the four basic operations, i.e. addition, subtraction, division and multiplication.
2. Written calculations should then be examined.

Praxis

Tests of apraxia can be divided in the following way:

1. Region of the body: limb vs orobuccal.
2. Meaningful vs meaningless (see Figure 5.4).

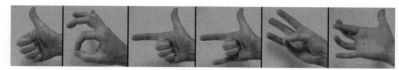

Fig. 5.4 A sequence of hand positions helpful in testing for apraxia.

3. For meaningful gestures: to command ("show me how to use a tooth-brush") vs by imitation.

4. With and without the real object.

Virtually all aphasic patients are impaired on miming to command, but performance often improves when imitating the examiner. A common error is the use of 'body-part-as-object', so that, for instance, when miming the use of a toothbrush, the forefinger substitutes as a brush, or when showing how to use a pair of scissors, the patient uses the index and middle fingers. The majority of apraxia patients perform meaningless gestures very poorly, and are worse at gesturing to command compared to copying or using real objects. A schedule for examining buccofacial and limb gestures is shown on p. 181.

Right Hemisphere Functions

Functions associated with the (for right-handers) non-dominant right hemisphere are:

A. Personal neglect
   • Denial of the existence of one side
   • Denial of hemiplegia (anosagnosia)
   • Unconcern about deficit (anosodiaphoria)

B. Sensory neglect
   • Visual, auditory and tactile neglect
   • Sensory extinction to simultaneous bilateral stimulation

C. Extrapersonal (hemispatial) neglect
   • Freehand copying of symmetrical representational drawings (for example, a clock-face, a double-headed daisy, etc.)
   • Visual search tests (for example, star cancellation)
   • Line bisection

D. Neglect dyslexia and dysgraphia
   • Line/page and word-based tests of reading and writing

E. Dressing apraxia

F. Visuo-spatial and constructional ability

G. Complex visuo-perceptual abilities and the agnosias

- Visual object agnosia
- Prosopagnosia

Personal neglect

Many patients with acute left hemiplegia do not realize that they are paralysed, and some frankly deny their deficit even when specifically challenged. This type of deficit is overlooked because examiners take it for granted that hemiplegic patients are aware that they are paralysed down one side. To detect these disorders it is necessary to question all stroke patients about their deficits and to compare their subjective assessments with objective findings. The following hierarchy of denial phenomena can be applied:

1. Denial of the existence of one side, sometimes accompanied by somatic delusions, such as that of the possession of three arms.

2. Denial of hemiplegia, but not of the existence of the affected part (anosagnosia).

3. Realization of hemiplegia, but with an underplaying of its severity and the resultant disability (anosodiaphoria).

Manifestations of personal (bodily) neglect

Personal neglect may be apparent because patients fail to groom one side of their head or shave one half of their face. Occasionally they have difficulty in dressing one side, or bump into objects on one side—usually the left. Head and eye deviation away from the neglected side (towards the lesion) implies damage to the frontal eye fields, and is a poor prognostic sign.

Sensory neglect

Patients with severe neglect may consistently ignore sensory inputs from the side contralateral to the side of their brain lesion. This usually occurs with right-sided lesions, so that the stimuli to the left are ignored. The following modalities should be tested.

Visual: The patient may ignore all visual stimuli to the contralateral side; if severe, this may be impossible to distinguish from hemianopia.

Auditory: The patient appears not to hear sounds to one side, and ignores visitors seated on that side of the bed.

Tactile: The patient ignores all sensory inputs from the affected side.

Sensory extinction to bilateral simultaneous stimulation is seen when the patient responds when stimuli (visual, auditory, or tactile) are presented to one side, but when simultaneously stimulated from both sides consistently ignores the neglected side.

Extrapersonal (hemispatial) neglect

Neglect of one half of space is fairly common after damage to either hemisphere; but persistent severe hemispatial neglect is seen only after right-sided damage. The following tests can be used to detect neglect phenomena.

1. *Freehand copying of representational drawings.* Items such as a clock-face, a flower-head or a house are conventionally used because they are two-dimensional and symmetrical. Drawing a clock-face is included in the ACE-R with a scoring scheme of 0–5: 1 for the circle; 1–2 for the numbers and their correct positioning and 1–2 for the hand settings (examples are given in Chapter 7). Another clinically useful drawing, a two-headed daisy in a plant pot, has proved to be very useful in screening patients for unilateral neglect. Samples are shown below. It can be seen that patients with neglect omit or fail to complete one side (see Figure 5.5). If asked to copy an array

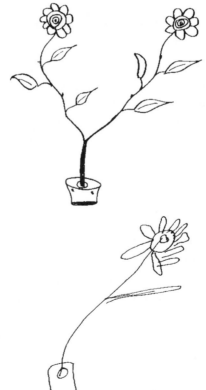

Fig. 5.5 Unilateral visual neglect: a right hemisphere stroke patient's attempt at copying the double-headed daisy, showing classic neglect of the left side. Provided by Dr Peter Halligan.

of items (for example, a house, a tree, and a man) they complete only one half of each item (see Figure 5.6). This phenomenon, referred to as **object-centred neglect**, demonstrates that the deficit is not a general neglect of the left half of space, but rather a specific defect in reconstructing the internal representation of individual objects.

2. *Visual search tasks*. Tests that require the subject to search a visual array for target shapes or letters are probably the most sensitive for detecting mild visual neglect. A recently devised version uses a mixture of words, letters and stars of various sizes scattered randomly across a sheet of A4 paper. The subject is asked to cross out all the small stars (see Appendix). An alternative version uses short lines at various angles scattered across a page. The subject is asked to cross out each of the lines.

3. *Line bisection*. Another traditional test of hemispatial neglect is to get the patient to mark the half-way point of lines of varying length. Patients with neglect consistently bisect the lines to the right of the mid-point.

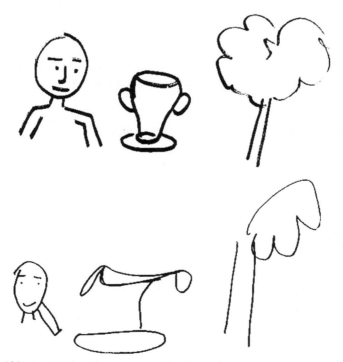

Fig. 5.6 Object-centred neglect: an example of a neglect patient's copy of three items in a single array. Provided by Dr Peter Halligan.

The degree of displacement is directly proportional to the length of the line used, so that the phenomenon is easier to detect using longer lines.

Neglect dyslexia and dysgraphia

These conditions are almost invariably associated with right-sided brain damage. Neglect dyslexia may affect lines of text or individual words. In the former, the patient omits the initial (left) part of each line, so that he or she reads only part of the text, rendering it nonsense. In the written equivalent, the patient writes on the right half of the page, and often leaves a progressively widening margin.

In word-based dyslexia, errors occur on reading the initial letters of words, which may be omissions (ISLAND to LAND) or substitutions (GRANT for PLANT). Word-based neglect dysgraphia causes the same type of errors, but in writing.

These syndromes are usually noted during language testing. But patients with other phenomena of neglect should be asked specifically to read a section of text from any book or magazine with wide columns. The word-list previously suggested for checking reading and writing should also detect word-based neglect dyslexia and dysgraphia.

Dressing apraxia

This is best detected by questioning family members or nursing staff. It may be observed on the ward. If there is any suggestion of dressing difficulty, a good test is to observe the patient putting on a shirt/blouse which has been turned inside out.

Visuo-spatial and constructional ability

Disorders of constructional ability are best detected by getting the patient to copy 3-D drawings, such as a wire cube, or a complex 2-D shape, such as the interlocking pentagons which form part of the Mini-Mental State Examination even patients with quite severe impairment of constructional skills may be able to copy simpler shapes, such as a Greek cross (Figure 5.7).

For a more stringent and quantitative test the Rey–Osterrieth Complex Figure Test is recommended, since the patient's copy can be scored using standard criteria (Figure 5.8). Delayed recall of the figure, usually after 30–40 min, can also be used as a measure of non-verbal memory.

Other formal tests for visuo-spatial and constructional abilities include:

- Block design from the WAIS
- Benton Line Orientation Test
- Components of the Visual Object and Space Perception (VOSP) battery

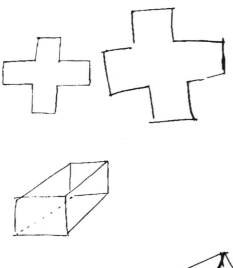

Fig. 5.7 Copy of a Greek cross and cube by a patient with a right-sided lesion, showing preservation of simple drawing but an inability to copy the 3-D cube.

Complex visuo-perceptual abilities and the agnosias

Deficits in object and face recognition are difficult to assess at the bedside without special test materials; but if there are clues that some form of agnosia may be present the following relatively simple tasks can be employed.

A. Object recognition

- Description of visually presented objects
- Matching objects in arrays
- Copying of drawings of objects
- Object matching
- Verbal knowledge of objects
- Tactile naming
- Formal tests: components of the VOSP (see Appendix)

B. Prosopagnosia

- Face description
- Face recognition and naming
- Face matching

- Verbal knowledge of misnamed persons
- Identification from voice, gait, etc.

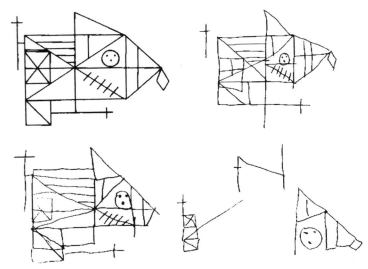

Fig. 5.8 The Rey–Osterrieth Complex Figure (upper left) and the copies of three patients with mild (upper right), moderate (lower left), and severe (lower right) impairment of constructional abilities.

Visual object agnosia

If the patient is unable to recognize simple objects or pictures despite good visual acuity and intact language abilities, a form of visual agnosia should be suspected.

In **apperceptual visual agnosia**, there is a breakdown at the stage of perceptual analysis, so that the patient is unable to describe the visually presented item and to match it with identical items. Patients' copies of drawings will be slow and fragmented, and identification of real objects is better than that of photographs or of line-drawings. Knowledge of the unidentified objects is preserved when tested verbally, and patients can identify objects by touch (see p. 86).

In **associative visual agnosia** the perceptual stages of object recognition are preserved, but patients are unable to make sense of the visual information; object description and matching are normal, and they can copy line drawings. In most cases, the deficit represents a loss of semantic knowledge (see p. 87). This causes an inability to name or identify items presented by any sensory modality, and a loss of verbal knowledge about the same items when asked probing questions (see Table 5.6).

Table 5.6 Differentiating the forms of visual agnosia

	Apperceptive	Associative
Object feature description	✕	✓
Visual identification	✕	✕
Copying line drawings	✕	✓
Object matching	✕	✓
Object knowledge (from name)	✓	✕
Tactile naming	✓	✕

✕, affected; ✓, spared.

Object feature description denotes the ability to describe the shape, outline, surface features, and colour of the presented object or picture.

Visual identification denotes the ability to recognize accurately the attributes of the visually presented stimulus even if unable to produce the name (for example, 'It's one of these things used by doctors to listen to your heart.').

Copying line drawings is tested by asking the patient to copy drawings of representational items such as a flower, a bicycle, a house, etc.

Object matching denotes the ability to match identical objects or pictures of objects. To test this it is necessary to use an array of items or pictures, two of which are identical. The patient is asked to point to the two items that are the same.

Object knowledge means the ability to generate accurate verbal descriptions when given the name of objects which the patient cannot identify visually ('what is a stethoscope?' etc.).

Tactile naming is tested by getting the patient to name objects by palpation with the eyes closed.

Prosopagnosia

Patients with severe deficits in visual analysis causing apperceptive agnosia are invariably impaired at recognizing faces. The syndrome of prosopagnosia is a specific form of associative agnosia in which visual perception of faces, and hence the ability to describe and match faces, is preserved, but there is a disorder of face recognition and identification. In suspected cases the following functions should be assessed.

1. *Face description*: the ability to analyse and describe constituent facial features such as age and sex and expressions is preserved.

2. *Face recognition and naming*: is severely defective.

3. *Face matching*: the ability to match together identical faces or portrait photographs should also be preserved.

4. *Knowledge of misnamed persons*: in classic (post-stroke) prosopagnosia there is retention of knowledge about famous people, friends and relatives, despite the inability to name them from photographs. In semantic dementia the deficit is cross-modal with a loss of knowledge about famous personalities whether tested using photographs or names.

5. *Identification* from voice, gait and dress is preserved in classic prosopagnosia.

Chapter 6

Standardized Mental Test Schedules: Their Uses and Abuses

Introduction

A large number of mental test schedules have been used over the years, which range in complexity from the 10-item Hodgkinson Mental Test, which takes only moments to complete, to the much more complex Dementia Rating Scale (DRS), which takes 30 min or more to administer. For practical purposes, however, such tests can be divided into two broad groups: (i) the brief schedules that can easily be used in the clinic, or at the bedside, and do not require specialized equipment or training, and (ii) the more elaborate scales, which are used largely, at least at present, in research studies, and require the purchase of test materials and some training in their administration. The Addenbrooke's Cognitive Examination (ACE) was developed in an attempt to bridge this divide and to provide a test with greater sensitivity to early cognitive decline than the Mini-Mental State Examination (MMSE) and which could also differentiate between different brain diseases. Chapter 7 describes in detail the revised version of the ACE with instructions on administration and scoring plus suggestions for supplementary testing in selected cases.

The remainder of this chapter covers possible alternative cognitive screening instruments. Because of the plethora of potential tests, I have chosen to describe three of the most commonly used brief assessment schedules: the MMSE, the Information–Memory–Concentration (IMC) Test, and the 10-item Hodgkinson Mental Test, which is derived from the IMC Test; plus two longer tests, which are widely used in dementia research: the Mattis Dementia Rating Scale (DRS) and the Cambridge Cognitive Examination—Revised (CAMCOG-R). Finally I have also included a description of the Alzheimer's Disease Assessment Scale (ADAS-Cog) since it has been used widely in drug evaluation studies.

All schedules have limitations and are open to abuses; but this applies particularly to the shorter tests. They are undoubtedly useful for screening large populations, since they have good inter-rater reliability and fairly well-established normative data; but the results must be interpreted with caution when applied to individual patients and they are of very limited application in a Memory or Cognitive Disorder Clinic. A number of general points deserve consideration before each test is described.

All the schedules sample a number of different areas of cognitive ability (for example, attention/concentration, memory, language, visuo-spatial abilities, etc.); hence failure can be due to various combinations of cognitive impairment. A low score may reflect appalling performance in one domain only, or slight impairment across all the domains evaluated. As a practical example, consider a score of 27 out of 30 on the MMSE. This could be due to a loss of all three recall points in the memory subset, or a loss of one point from each of three of the five subsets, orientation, attention, memory (registration and recall), language or visuo-spatial. Both patterns produce the same total score, but the former is clearly much more significant. This illustrates how essential it is to consider the profile of performance on these tests, and not just the overall total score.

It should be emphasized that all the schedules were developed with a view to quantifying the cognitive failings in elderly subjects with dementia and/or delirium. They may, with certain provisos, be reliable measures in these situations; but this does not mean that they can be applied generally to patients with all types of cognitive impairment, both focal and general, acute and chronic. Of particular note is their insensitivity to circumscribed cognitive deficits. This is exemplified in patients with extensive right hemisphere lesions, who may have major visuo-spatial and perceptual deficits, but score almost perfectly on any of the mental test schedules under consideration (except the ACE-R). They are also notoriously insensitive to frontal lobe disorders, and patients with disabling and profound deficits in 'executive' and social functions typically perform normally, even on the more extensive screening batteries.

It should also be realized that the normative values and 'cut-off' levels generally applied in these tests veer towards specificity, rather than sensitivity, in dementia. A score below the cut-off of 24 on the MMSE (in the absence of features of delirium) is a fairly good marker of dementia. However, many patients with early Alzheimer's disease score above this cut-off, particularly if they are young and of superior background intellectual ability.

This brings up the important question of considering background demographic features, which are likely to affect performance. Age, education and socio-economic status are the most important variables. Ethnic group and first language should also be considered. These factors are additive, so that the lower limit of normal for an elderly person with only a few years of education is radically different to that of a young, highly educated professional.

These points will be discussed further in relation to the test schedules under consideration.

Mini-Mental State Examination (MMSE)

Instructions: Record response to each question.

Domain tested	Score

Orientation

+ Year, month, day, date, season ___/5
+ Country, county (district), town, hospital, ward (room) ___/5

Registration (memory)

+ Examiner names three objects (e.g. lemon, key, ball).
  Patient asked to repeat three names ___/3

Attention

+ Subtract 7 from 100, then repeat from result, etc.
  Stop after five trials: 100, 93, 86, 79, 72, 65 (do not correct if errors made)
  (alternative if unable to perform serial subtraction: spell 'world' backwards: D L R O W).
  Score the best performance on either task ___/5

Recall (memory)

+ Ask for the names of the three objects learned earlier. ___/3

Language

+ Name a pencil and a watch. ___/2
+ Repeat 'No ifs, ands, or buts'. ___/1
+ Give a three-stage command. Score one for each stage
  (e.g. 'Take this piece of paper in your right hand, fold it in half,
  and place it on the chair next to you.'). ___/3
+ Ask patient to read and obey a written command on a piece of
  paper that states:
  'Close your eyes.' ___/1
+ Ask patient to write a sentence. Score if it is sensible, and has a
  subject and a verb. ___/1

Copying

+ Ask patient to copy intersecting pentagons (Figure 6.1). ___/1

Total score ___/30

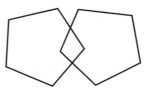

Fig. 6.1 Overlapping pentagons from the Mini-Mental State Examination.

The MMSE, designed by Folstein and colleagues from Baltimore in the 1970s, is the most widely used and studied screening measure of cognitive impairment. It has the advantages of brevity, ease of administration, and high inter-rater reliability. It can be easily incorporated into routine clinical practice, and provides a good rough-and-ready screening test for dementia and delirium. It is also of practical value in monitoring progression in these disorders. It is not useful, however, for the detection of mild cognitive impairment, focal deficits (amnesia, aphasia, visuo-spatial disorders etc.), and is insensitive to frontal lobe disorders.

A score of less than 24 was initially suggested for distinguishing between impaired and normal subjects, respectively, with a reasonably high degree of specificity and sensitivity. However, these values were derived from screening elderly hospitalized patients with delirium or fairly advanced degrees of dementia, not outpatients with mild disease. Mild cases with early, but clinically definite, Alzheimer's disease score above this level. It has also been clearly established that the MMSE is quite vulnerable to the effects of age, education and socio-economic status. The following age-related cut-offs have been proposed:

40s: 29/30

50s: 28/30

60s: 28/30

70s: 28/30

80s: 26/30

Further adjustments are required for educational level, especially in the older age-groups. For subjects aged over 70 years who left school before the age of 15 (i.e. those with less than 10 years of education), a score of up to three less than the age-related score given above is acceptable as normal.

There are also difficulties with scoring the attentional subtest. The authors of the MMSE originally suggested that the spelling of the word WORLD backwards should be given to those unable to perform serial subtraction. However, this instruction is rather loose, and leads to confusion. We have tended to administer serial sevens, and if any errors occur we give subjects the task of spelling WORLD backwards. The score is then taken as the best performance on either of these two. Other authors have opted to give either the serial sevens or the WORLD backward test to each subject.

The subtests most useful in detecting early Alzheimer's disease are the recall of the three items, followed by orientation and drawing, although we have shown that the MMSE is far less sensitive than the ACE for screening in a memory clinic setting. The language tests are the least sensitive component of the MMSE. In Huntington's disease and other forms of subcortical dementia, such as progressive supranuclear palsy (PSP), the attentional subtests are those most vulnerable to disease, but again, the MMSE lacks sensitivity. The MMSE is susceptible to 'floor effects' in severely demented cases. That is to say, once patients reach a fairly advanced stage of disease they tend to score very few points, and beyond this progression cannot be assessed.

Information–Memory–Concentration (IMC) Test: American Modification by Fuld

Instructions: One point for each correct answer unless otherwise indicated.

Domain tested	Score
Information	
◆ Name	—
◆ Age	—
◆ Time (hour)	—
◆ Time of day	—
◆ Day of week	—
◆ Date	—
◆ Month	—
◆ Season	—
◆ Year	—
◆ Place: name	—
street	—
town	—
◆ Type of place (for example, home, hospital, etc.)	—
Total	__/13

Memory (NB: Administer name and address at this stage)

Personal

◆ Date of birth

◆ Place of birth

- School attended
- Occupation
- Mother's first name   Total   __/5

Non-personal

- Date of First World War: 1914–1918 (half point if either date within 3 years)
- Date of Second World War: 1939–1945 (half point if either date within 3 years)
- President (or Prime Minister)
- Past President (or past Prime Minister)   Total   __/4

Five-minute recall of name and address (score 0–5 points)

e.g. Mr John Brown

    42 West Street

    Gateshead   Total   __/5

Concentration (all scored 0–1–2)

- Months of the year backwards
- Counting 1–20
- Counting 20–1   Total   __/6

Maximum error score = 33

The IMC Test, first published in 1968 as part of the Blessed Dementia Rating Scale, has been widely used and adapted since. The version shown is the American adaptation by Fuld, which has been well validated. The popularity of the IMC Test owes much to the fact that it remains virtually the only scale for which performance has been correlated with neuropathological parameters of severity in Alzheimer's disease, namely density of plaques and levels of choline acetyltransferase in post-mortem brains.

Its advantages, uses and limitations are, in principle, the same as those of the MMSE, although the effects of age, education and socio-economic status on it have not been as thoroughly evaluated. Because of the heavy weighting towards memory it is perhaps more sensitive to the early changes of Alzheimer's disease than the MMSE, although a number of studies have shown that performance on the two tests is closely correlated. Unlike other mental test schedules, the IMC Test is scored as the total number of errors, with a maximum of 33 in the Fuld version shown. More than four errors has been considered abnormal. But the cut-off should certainly be higher for the very elderly with low educational attainment, and should perhaps be even lower for young professionals.

Because of the emphasis on orientation and attentional tasks it is theoretically a good initial screening tool for acute confusional states (delirium), although this has not been well studied.

Hodgkinson Mental Test

Instructions: Score one point for each question answered correctly.

Question	Score
◆ Age of patient	__
◆ Time (to nearest hour)	__
◆ Address given, for recall at end of test: 42 West Street	__
◆ Name of hospital (*or* area of town if at home)	__
◆ Year	__
◆ Date of birth of patient	__
◆ Month	__
◆ Years of First World War	__
◆ Name of Monarch (President in USA)	__
◆ Count backwards from 20 to 1 (no errors allowed, but may correct self)	__
Total	__/10

Derived from the Blessed Information–Concentration–Memory Test, this test has been fairly widely used and validated for use with the elderly, but has not been studied to anything like the extent of the MMSE. The major, and arguably the only, point in its favour is its extreme brevity. An overall score of 6/10 or less is said to be abnormal in the elderly. Values for younger patients have not been established. Clearly not all questions are equivalent, and, as with other schedules, the profile of scores should be considered. It has no major advantages over the MMSE and IMC Test. If a brief screening schedule is required for general clinical use, I would favour one of those tests.

Mattis Dementia Rating Scale (DRS)

(Published by Psychological Assessment Resources)

DRS subtests	Score
Attention subtest	
Digit span (forwards and backward)	__/8
Two-step commands	__/2

One-step commands		__/4
Imitation of commands		__/4
Counting As		__/6
Counting randomly arranged As		__/5
Reading a word list		__/4
Matching figures		__/4
	Total	__/37

Initiation subtest

Fluency for supermarket items		__/20
Fluency for clothing items		__/8
Verbal repetition (e.g. bee, key, gee)		__/2
Double alternating movements		__/3
Graphomotor (copy alternating figures)		__/4
	Total	__/37

Construction subtest

Copy geometrical designs		__/6
	Total	__/6

Conceptualization subtest

Similarities		__/8
Inductive reasoning		__/3
Detection of different item		__/3
Multiple-choice similarities		__/8
Identities and oddities		__/16
Create a sentence		__/1
	Total	__/39

Memory subtest

Recall a sentence (I)		__/4
Recall a self-generated sentence (II)		__/3
Orientation (e.g. date, place)		__/9
Verbal recognition		__/5
Figure recognition		__/4
	Total	__/25
	Total score	__/144

Originally designed by Mattis for use in a prospective study of dementia, the DRS assesses a fairly wide range of cognitive abilities, and contains a sufficient number of less-demanding items such that valid and reliable information can be obtained in more severely demented subjects. Its principal use is in research, particularly that involving longitudinal studies of demented patients or the comparison of patients with different pathologies.

It is easy to administer and score. The first four sections—attention, initiation, construction, and conceptualization—are graded in difficulty, and contain screening tests at the beginning. If these are passed, the remainder of the section need not be administered. The final memory section is given to all subjects. Approximately 20–40 min are required to administer it to demented patients, depending upon their level of impairment. Test–retest reliability is excellent and it has good construct validity compared to formal neuropsychological evaluation as the 'gold standard'.

Normal elderly subjects perform well on the DRS. The mean total score in early studies ranged from 137 to 140. Our own early experience, together with that of the San Diego Alzheimer's disease research group, suggested a cut-off of 132 for separating impaired from normal subjects. Since the publication of the first edition of this book, a number of studies have been published showing the predicted effects of age, education and socio-economic status. For instance, a study from Brazil suggested that a cut-off score of 122 produced around 90% sensitivity and specificity for the diagnosis of dementia, but age and schooling level had a significant effect on the scores. A similar study from North America recommended that a cut-off of 123 was required in a broader population to produce acceptable sensitivity and specificity values.

The DRS has been most widely used in patients with Alzheimer's disease. It is more sensitive to early disease than the brief scales discussed above, and shows less marked floor effects. It may also be helpful in distinguishing between different dementing illnesses. The memory section is most sensitive to Alzheimer's whereas patients with Huntington's disease are most impaired on the initiation subtest. We have recently compared performance on the DRS and ACE of large groups of patients with Alzheimer's disease, PSP, corticobasal degeneration (CBD) and multiple system atrophy (MSA). Each disorder produced a distinctive profile which was apparent on both the ACE and the DRS. Figure 6.2 shows the proportion of cases demonstrating impairment on each subtest. It can be seen that the ACE was more sensitive overall, that MSA patients showed least impairment while those with CBD showed global deficits compared with the much more selective profiles demonstrated in AD and PSP.

It should also be noted that the DRS provides a broad test of the distributed cognitive functions (attention, memory, and abstraction/conceptualization),

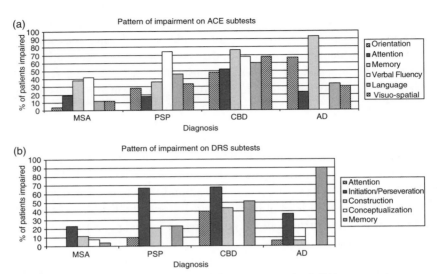

Fig. 6.2 Proportion of patients with multiple system atrophy (MSA), progressive supranuclear palsy (PSP), corticobasal degeneration (CBD) and Alzheimer's disease (AD) showing impairment on subtests of (a) Addenbrooke's Cognitive Examination (ACE) and (b) Dementia Rating Scale (DRS).

but includes virtually no assessment of localized functions, especially language. This is of relevance when attempting to screen for semantic dementia and progressive non-fluent aphasia.

Cambridge Cognitive Examination: CAMCOG

(Published by Cambridge University Press)

CAMCOG-R subtests		**Scores**
Orientation		
Time—day, date, month, year, season		
Place—county, town, street, floor, place	Total	__/10
Language		
Comprehension		
Expression: naming of objects and pictures, definitions		
Verbal fluency (animals)		
Repetition of "no ifs, ands, or buts"		
Reading comprehension		
	Total	__/30

Memory

Registration and recall of three items from MMSE

Recall and recognition of pictures

Remote and recent information retrieval

| | Total | __/27 |

Attention and caluclation

Counting backwards and serial 7s

| | Total | __/9 |

Praxis

Copying and drawing (pentagons, spiral, house, clock)

Actions to command

Writing—spontaneous and to dictation

| | Total | __/12 |

Abstract thinking

Similarities

| | Total | __/8 |

Perception

Visual recognition, unusual views and famous people naming

| | Total | __/9 |
| | Total score | __/105 |

Additional tasks in CAMCOG-R

Ideational fluency

Visual reasoning

| | Total | __/14 |
| | Overall grand score | __/119 |

The CAMCOG forms part of a standardized psychiatric assessment schedule, CAMDEX (Cambridge Examination for Mental Disorders of the Elderly), devised by Roth and colleagues and published by Cambridge University Press (1988). CAMDEX was designed specifically for use in elderly people with the diagnosis of dementia and was later revised as CAMDEX-R (1998). It includes: a structured psychiatric interview with the patient; a relative or other informant interview; a brief physical examination; and a neuropsychological test battery, CAMCOG-R.

CAMCOG-R assesses a wider range of cognitive functions, both distributed (attention, memory, abstraction) and localized (language, praxis, etc.), than any other standardized schedule. It incorporates both the MMSE and the IMC within the battery. The CAMCOG-R also includes two additional tests of executive function (ideational fluency—uses of a bottle—and a visual reasoning test similar to Raven's matrices). The average administration time is 20–40 min, depending on the degree of impairment. The maximum overall score is 105. A cut-off of 80 was found to discriminate between demented and normal subjects, respectively, on the original validation studies with a high degree of specificity and sensitivity. Further work has shown that, in keeping with other mental test schedules, the normal range varies considerably with age, and age-appropriate normative values are now available. For instance, in a large community sample the 10th centile score was shown to fall from 85 for subjects aged 60–69 years to 65 for those aged 85–89 years.

CAMCOG has been used extensively in community-based studies of dementia around Europe, and is the best-validated and normed of the longer mental test batteries. The CAMCOG-R was used in a multinational harmonization project (EURO-HARPID) and has been translated for use around Europe. The value of either CAMCOG or CAMCOG-R in distinguishing between patients with various types of dementia is less well established, but recent work has shown that it is sensitive to cognitive dysfunction in Parkinson's disease and post-stroke dementia. Evidence is also emerging to suggest that it can reveal distinct profiles in AD and dementia with Lewy bodies (DLB).

In comparison with the DRS, CAMCOG is likely to be more sensitive to mild degrees of dementia, and should be better at detecting patients with predominantly language or visuo-spatial dysfunction as the DRS contains no language tests and only a limited assessment of drawing ability. A disadvantage of CAMCOG is the relative lack of very easy items, so that it is unlikely to be as valuable as the DRS for monitoring progress in patients with moderately severe dementia.

Alzheimer's Disease Assessment Scale (ADAS)

The ADAS-Cognitive subscale (ADAS-Cog) was the primary cognitive outcome measure in the first clinical trials of drugs for the treatment of dementia and has subsequently become one of the two primary outcome measures required by the US Food and Drug Administration authority for the licensing of new drugs. Numerous translations are available. It was designed by Rosen and her colleagues to test three cognitive domains: memory, language and praxis. It has a mixture of objective assessments, such as word list learning and naming, together with observer-rated assessments of language and praxis. It contains the following subscores.

Orientation

Total possible errors _____/8

Language ability

Naming objects and fingers

Observer-rated comprehension of spoken language, expressive language and word finding

Total possible errors _____/25

Memory

Word-list learning, recall and recognition

Recall of test instructions

Total possible errors _____/27

Praxis

Consisting of constructional praxis (copying geometric figures) and ideational praxis (preparing envelope to send to oneself)

Total possible errors _____/10

Overall grand score/errors _____/70

The ADAS score is based upon the number of errors ranging from 0 to 70 with the highest scores indicating the greatest impairment. It takes 30–35 min to administer. As with other similar tests, age and education have a significant effect on ADAS-Cog performance. Inter-rater reliability is good. It has been used extensively in drug trials but we have limited experience in Cambridge. It has very doubtful sensitivity to other dementia syndromes and its usefulness in screening for mild cognitive impairment is doubtful.

Chapter 7

The Addenbrooke's Cognitive Examination—Revised and Supplementary Test Suggestions

This chapter describes the use of the revised version of the Addenbrooke's Cognitive Examination: ACE-R. The original test was developed in our clinics in the 1990s and was shown to be sensitive to early Alzheimer's disease (AD) and to differentiate AD from frontotemporal dementia (FTD). In addition it was shown to be useful in the separation of organic brain disease from psychiatric states, and in the detection of cognitive dysfunction associated with the parkinsonian syndromes of progressive supranuclear palsy (PSP), corticobasal degeneration (CBD) and multiple system atrophy (MSA) (for references to the ACE see selected further reading at end of book). The main weaknesses were the imbalance across domains (especially the limited range of visuo-spatial/perceptual tasks), the insensitivity of the naming component and the difficulty in translation of certain components. Another goal in developing the ACE-R was to have a version with clearer cognitive subtest scores. The ACE-R went through multiple prototypes before arriving at the final version. This chapter describes the ACE-R together with scoring criteria and normative data followed by suggestions for 'add-on' bedside tasks that test areas not well covered by the ACE-R.

THE ADDENBROOKE'S COGNITIVE EXAMINATION—ACE-R
Revised Version A (2005)

Name:	Date of testing: ____/____/____
Date of birth:	Tester's name: _____
Hospital no.:	Age at leaving full-time education: _____
	Occupation: _____
	Handedness: _____
Addressograph	

ORIENTATION

➤ Ask: What is the	Day	Date	Month	Year	Season	[Score 0–5]

➤ Ask: Which	Building	Floor	Town	County	Country	[Score 0–5]

REGISTRATION

➤ Tell: 'I'm going to give you three words and I'd like you to repeat after me: lemon, key and ball.' After subject repeats, say 'Try to remember them because I'm going to ask you later.' Score *only* the first trial (repeat 3 times if necessary).

[Score 0–5]

Register number of trials _____

ATTENTION & CONCENTRATION

➤ Ask the subject: 'Could you take 7 away from 100?' After the subject responds, ask him or her to take away another 7 to a total of 5 subtractions. If subject makes a mistake, carry on and check the subsequent answer (i.e. 93, 84, 77, 70, 63–score 4). Stop after five subtractions (93, 86, 79, 72, 65 ____ ____ ____

____ ____

[Score 0–5]

(for the best performed task)

➤ Ask: 'Could you please spell **WORLD** for me?' Then ask him/her to spell it backwards:

____ ____ ____ ____ ____

MEMORY — Recall

➤ Ask: 'Which 3 words did I asked you to repeat and remember?'   [Score 0–3]

____ ____ ____

MEMORY — Anterograde Memory

➤ Tell: 'I'm going to give you a name and address and I'd like you to repeat after me. We'll be doing that 3 times, so you have a chance to learn it. I'll be asking you later.'   [Score 0–7]

Score only the third trial

	1st Trial	2nd Trial	3rd Trial	
Harry Barnes	_ _	_ _	_ _	
73 Orchard Close	_ _ _	_ _ _	_ _ _	
Kingsbridge	_	_	_	
Devon	_	_	_	

MEMORY — Retrograde Memory

➤ Name of current Prime Minister _____   [Score 0–4]

➤ Name of the woman who was Prime Minister _____

➤ Name of the USA president _____

➤ Name of the USA president who was assassinated _____

VERBAL FLUENCY — Letter 'P' and animals

➤ Letters

Say: 'I'm going to give you a letter of the alphabet and I'd like you to generate as many words as you can beginning with that letter, but not names of people or places. Are you ready? You've got a minute for that and the letter is letter P.'   [Score 0–7]

				>17	7
				14–17	6
				11–13	5
				8–10	4
				6–7	3
				4–5	2
				2–3	1
				<2	0
				total	correct

➤ **Animals** [Score 0–7]

Say: 'Now can you name as many animals as possible, beginning with any letter'

					>21	7
					17–21	6
					14–16	5
					11–13	4
					9–10	3
					7–8	2
					5–6	1
					<5	0
					total	correct

LANGUAGE — Comprehension

➤ Show written instruction: [Score 0–1]

Close your eyes

➤ 3 stage command: [Score 0–3]

'Take the paper in your right hand. Fold the paper in half. Put the paper on the floor.'

LANGUAGE — Writing

➤ Ask the subject to make up a sentence and write it in the space below: [Score 0–1]

Score 1 if sentence contains a subject and a verb (see guide for examples)

LANGUAGE — Repetition

➤ Ask the subject to repeat: **'hippopotamus'**; **'eccentricity'**; **'unintelligible'**; **'statistician'** [Score 0–2]

Score 2 if all correct; 1 if 3 correct; 0 if 2 or less.

➤ Ask the subject to repeat: **'Above, beyond and below'** [Score 0–1]

➤ Ask the subject to repeat: '**No ifs, ands or buts**'

[Score 0–1]

LANGUAGE — Naming

➤ Ask the subject to name the following pictures:

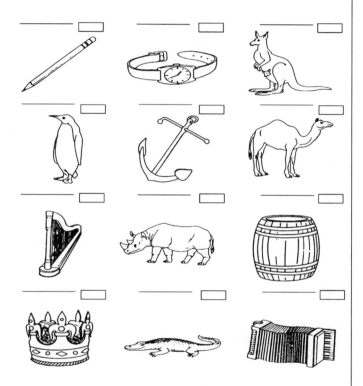

LANGUAGE — Comprehension

➤ Using the pictures above, ask the subject to:

[Score 0–4]

- ◆ Point to the one which is associated with the monarchy _____

- ◆ Point to the one which is a marsupial _____

- ◆ Point to the one which is found in the Antarctic _____

- ◆ Point to the one which has a nautical connection _____

LANGUAGE — Reading

➤ Ask the subject to read the following words: (Score 1 only if all correct)

[Score 0–1]

sew
pint
soot
dough
height

VISUOSPATIAL ABILITIES

➤ Overlapping pentagons: Ask the subject to copy this diagram:

[Score 0–1]

➤ Wire cube: Ask the subject to copy this drawing (for scoring, see instructions guide)

[Score 0–2]

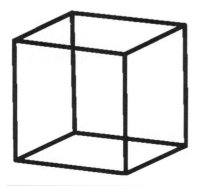

➤ Clock: Ask the subject to draw a clock face with numbers and the hands at ten past five. (For scoring see instructions guide: circle = 1, numbers = 2, hands = 2 if all correct) [Score 0–5]

PERCEPTUAL ABILITIES

➤ Ask the subject to count the dots without pointing them [Score 0–4]

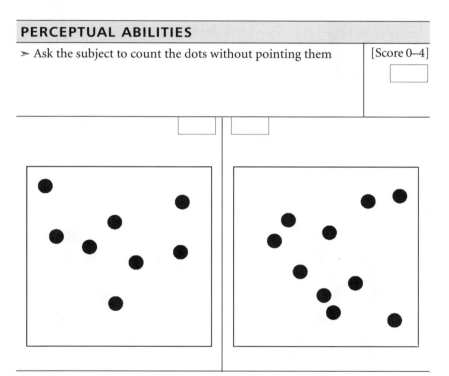

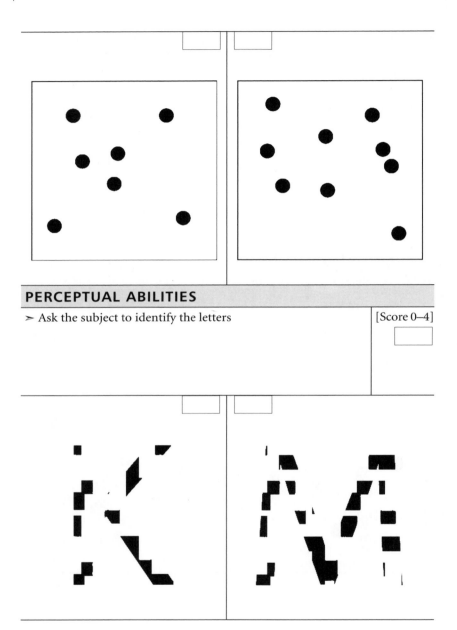

PERCEPTUAL ABILITIES

➤ Ask the subject to identify the letters   [Score 0–4]

RECALL

➤ Ask "Now tell me what you remember of that name and address we were repeating at the beginning"

		[Score 0–7]
Harry Barnes	....	
73 Orchard Close	....	
Kingsbridge	....	
Devon	....	

RECOGNITION

➤ This test should be done if subject failed to recall one or more items. If all items were recalled, skip the test and score 5. If only part is recalled start by ticking items recalled in the shaded column on the right hand side. Then test not-recalled items by telling 'Ok, I'll give you some hints: was the name X, Y or Z?' and so on. Each recognized item scores one point which is added to the point gained by recalling.

[Score 0–5]

Jerry Barnes		Harry Barnes		Harry Bradford		recalled	
Orchard Place		Oak Close		Orchard Close		recalled	
37		73		76		recalled	
Oakhampton		Kingsbridge		Dartington		recalled	
Devon		Dorset		Somerset		recalled	

General scores

MMSE	/30
ACE-R	/100

Subscores

Attention and Orientation	/18
Memory	/26
Fluency	/14
Language	/26
Visuo-spatial	/16

ADDENBROOKE'S COGNITIVE EXAMINATION — ACE-R

Administration and Scoring Guide — 2006

The ACE-R is a brief cognitive test that assesses five cognitive domains, namely attention/orientation, memory, verbal fluency, language and visuo-spatial abilities. Total score is 100, higher scores indicates better cognitive functioning.

Administration of the ACE-R takes, on average, 15 min.

These instructions have been designed in order to make the questions and their scoring clear for the tester. Please read them carefully before giving the test.

If possible, leave the scoring until the end of the session, since the participant will not be able to check whether the tester is ticking for correct answers or crossing for wrong ones. This might avoid anxiety, which can disturb the participant's performance on the test.

ORIENTATION — score 0 to 10

Ask the participant for the day, date, month, year and season. Score one point for each correct answer.

Ask the participant for the name of the hospital (or building), the floor (or room), the town, county and country. Score one point for each correct answer. Record responses. Allow mistakes for the date (+ or − 2 days). If assessing a participant at home, ask for the name of the place, i.e. name of the house e.g. "The Gables", and for the floor you might ask for the name of the room (kitchen, living room, etc.). If at a single storey health setting, ask about a local landmark. When the season is changing, e.g. at the end of August, and the participant says "autumn", ask them "could it be another season?". If answer is "summer", give one point, since the two seasons are in transition. Do not give one point if the answer is "winter" or "spring".

Seasons: spring — March, April, May; summer — June, July, August; autumn — September, October, November; winter — December, January, February.

REGISTRATION — score 0 to 3

Ask the participant to repeat and remember the words lemon, key, and ball. Speak slowly. Repeat them if necessary (maximum 3 times). Tell the participant that you will ask for this information later. Record the number of trials. Score the first attempt only.

ATTENTION & CONCENTRATION — score 0 to 5

Calculation: Ask the participant to subtract 7 from 100, record the answer, then ask them to subtract 7 from that, record the answer. Do this 5 times. If the participant makes a mistake, carry on and check subsequent answers for scoring. Record responses (example: 92, 85, 79, 72, 65, score 3).

Spelling: give this test if the participant makes a mistake on the calculation task. Start by asking the participant to spell "world". Then ask them to spell it backwards. Record responses.

Scoring for the spelling task:

- Score 1 point for each correct letter spelt. Correct sequence = D L R O W = 5 points

- Count one error for each omission, letter transposition (switching adjacent letters), insertion (inserting a new letter), or misplacement (moving W, O, R, L, D by more than one space).

Examples (score in parentheses):

	omission	transposition	insertion	misplacement
omission	DLOW (4)			
transposition	D**OL**W (3)	D**LOR**W (4)		
	omission	transposition	insertion	misplacement
insertion	DL**T**OW (3)	DLR**WWO** (3)	DLR**RR**OW(4)	
misplacement	LOW**D** (3)	LR**WOD** (3)	LR**WOWD** (3)	LROWD (4)

A response such as 'LRWWOD' has 3 errors (L and R are correct, for a score of 2). It includes transposition of the W and O, insertion of an extra W, and misplacement of the D. If the patient adds 1 or more of the same letter at the end of the word, count as one error (e.g. 'LDROWWW', would be 2 errors, 1 transposition and 1 addition).

Score one point for each correct calculation or letter spelt. Score only the better-performed one.

RECALL — score 0 to 3

Ask the participant to recall the words that you asked them to repeat and remember. Record responses. Score one point for each correct item.

Anterograde Memory — score 0 to 7

Instruct the participant: "I'm going to read you a name and address that I'd like you to repeat after me. We'll be doing that 3 times, so you have a chance to learn it.

I'll be asking you about it later." If the participant starts repeating along with you, ask them to wait until you give it in full.

Record responses for each trial. However, only the third score contributes to the ACE-R score (0–7 points).

Retrograde Memory — score 0 to 4

Ask the participant for the name of the current Prime Minister, the woman who was Prime Minister, the president of the USA and the president of the USA who was assassinated in the 1960s.

Score one point each. Allow answers like Blair, Thatcher, Bush, Kennedy. Do not accept answers like Maggie, ask for surname as well.

VERBAL FLUENCY — score 0 to 14

Letters — score 0 to 7

Instruct the participant: "I'm going to give you a letter of the alphabet and I'd like you to generate as many words as you can beginning with that letter, but not the names of people or places. Are you ready? You've got a minute and the letter is P."

Participant might repeat or perseverate words, e.g. pay, paid, pays. Record and count them for the overall total number of responses but do not consider them for the final score. In the same way, intrusions such as words beginning with other letters are recorded but not scored. Proper names (Peter, Peterborough) do not count. For plurals, e.g. pot, pots, total = 2, correct = 1. Use the table provided on the ACE-R sheet to obtain the final score for this test.

Animals — score 0 to 7

Instruct the participant: "Now can you name as many animals as possible, beginning with any letter?"

Participant might repeat words. Record and count them for the overall total number of responses, but they should not be considered for the final score. The participant may misunderstand and perseverate by naming animals beginning with "p". Repeat instructions during the 60 seconds if necessary.

If subject says, e.g. "fish", and later says "salmon" and "trout", count and record as 3 for "total" but do not accept "fish" as correct (count only 2 out of the 3, e.g. "salmon" and "trout"). However, if only the category is given, e.g. fish, with no specific exemplars, then count fish as 1 for total and final correct responses. The same applies to mammals, reptiles, birds, breeds of dog, insects, etc.

LANGUAGE — Comprehension — score 0 or 1

Comprehension (Close your eyes)

Instruct the participant: "Read this sentence and do as it says." If the participant reads sentence aloud but does not follow the instructions, score 0.

LANGUAGE — Comprehension — score 0 or 3

Comprehension (3-stage command)

Instruct the participant: "Take this paper in your right hand, fold it in half, and put it on the floor." Do not allow participant to take the paper before you have finished giving the complete instruction.

Score one point for each correct command, e.g. if participant takes the paper and puts it on the floor without folding, score 2; if participant takes the paper in their right hand, and folds it several times and leaves on the table, score 1.

LANGUAGE — Writing — score 0 or 1

Instruct the participant to write a sentence.

The sentence should contain a subject and a verb, and it should have a meaning.

Do not accept "Happy Birthday" or "Nice day" as a sentence. If participant has difficulty thinking of something to write, prompt gently with "What's the weather like today?"

LANGUAGE — Repetition — score 0 or 2

Ask the participant to repeat the words after you. Say one word at a time. Circle the words that were repeated incorrectly. Consider first attempt only for scoring. Record responses. Score 2 if all words are correct; 1 if 3 are correct; 0 if 2 or less are correct.

LANGUAGE — Repetition — score 0 or 2

Ask the participant to repeat each sentence. Do not accept partially correct repetitions, e.g. "no ifs and buts", "above below" as correct for scoring. Score one point for each sentence.

LANGUAGE — Naming — score 0 or 2

Naming (watch and pencil)

Ask the participant to name each picture. Correct answers: pencil; wristwatch or watch.

LANGUAGE — Naming — score 0 or 10

Naming (5 animals and 5 objects)

Ask the participant to name each picture. Correct answers: penguin; anchor; camel or dromedary; barrel or tub; crown; crocodile or alligator; harp; rhinoceros or rhino; kangaroo or wallaby; piano accordion, accordion or squeeze box. Score one point each.

LANGUAGE — Comprehension — score 0 or 4

Comprehension

Ask the participant to point to the pictures according to the statement read. Score one point each. Allow self-corrections.

LANGUAGE — Reading — score 0 or 1

Ask the participant to read the words aloud. Score one point only if all five words are correctly read. Record the mistakes using the phonetic alphabet if possible.

VISUO-SPATIAL ABILITIES — Overlapping Pentagons — score 0 or 1

The pentagons should clearly show 5 sides and the intersection.

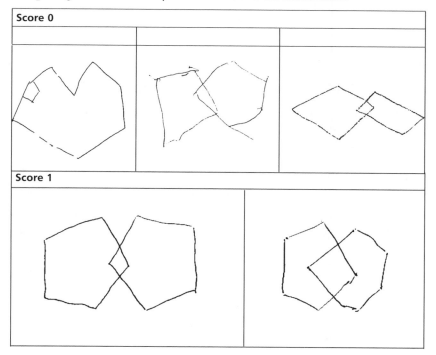

Score 0		

Score 1

VISUO-SPATIAL ABILITIES — Wire Cube — score 0 to 2

Cube should have 12 lines = score 2, even if the proportions are not perfect. A score of 1 is given if cube has fewer than 12 lines, but general cube shape is maintained. See examples below.

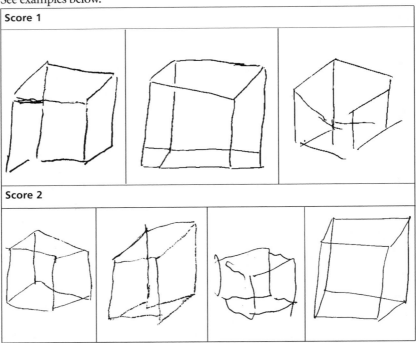

VISUO-SPATIAL ABILITIES — Clock — score 0 to 5

Ask the participant to draw a clock face with the numbers on it. When he/she has finished, ask them to put the hands at 'ten past five'.

Circle	1 point maximum if it is a reasonable circle
Numbers	2 points if all included and well distributed
	1 point if all included but poorly distributed
Hands	2 points if both hands are well drawn, different lengths and placed on correct numbers (you might ask which one is the small one and which is the big one)
	1point if both placed on the correct numbers but wrong lengths OR
	1 point if one hand is placed on the correct number and drawn with correct length OR
	1 point if only one hand is drawn and placed at the correct number i.e. 5 for 'ten past five'

Score 2	
Circle (1); one hand placed correctly (1)	Circle (1); all the numbers but not placed inside the circle (1)
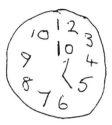	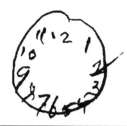

Score 3		
Circle (1); all the numbers but not proportionally distributed (1), one hand placed correctly (1)	Circle (1), all the numbers but not placed inside the circle (1), one hand place correctly (1)	Circle (1), note that numbers are not inside the circle and there are 2 number 10s (0), hands placed correctly
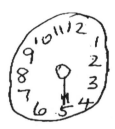	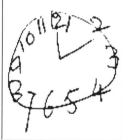	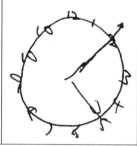

Score 4		
Circle (1); numbers proportionally distributed (2); one hand placed correctly (1)	Circle (1); all the numbers but not proportionally distributed (1); both hands placed correctely (2)	Circle (1); numbers proportionally distributed (2), one hand placed correctly (1)
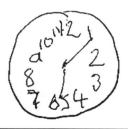	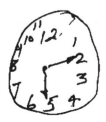	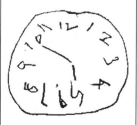

Score 5

Circle (1); numbers proportionally distributed on both halves of the clock face (2); hands placed correctly (2)

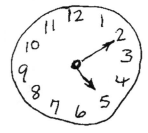

PERCEPTUAL ABILITIES — score 0 to 4

Counting dots

Participant is *not* allowed to point to the picture. Score one point for each correct answer.

Correct answers, from top left clockwise: 8, 10, 9 and 7.

PERCEPTUAL ABILITIES — score 0 to 4

Identifying letters

Participant is allowed to point to the picture. Score one point for each correct answer.

Correct answers, from top left clockwise: K, M, T and A.

RECALL — score 0 to 7

Recall

Say to the participant: "Now tell me what you remember of that name and address we were repeating at the beginning." Tick and score one point for each item recalled, using the score guide provided in the test.

Harry Barnes
73 Orchard Close
Kingsbridge
Devon

Example 1a

Harry Bond	1 + 0	
78 Orchard Close	0 + 1 + 1	
Kingsbury	0	
....	0	Score 3/7

Example 2a

Harry Barnes	$1 + 1$	
73 Kingsbridge Close	$1 + 0 + 1$	
....	0	
Devon	1	**Score 5/7**

Example 3a

Harry Bond	$1 + 0$	
33 Kingsbury Way	$0 + 0 + 0$	
Kingsbridge Close	$0 + 0$	
Cambridge	0	
Devon	1	**Score 2/7**

RECOGNITION — score 0 to 5

Recognition – only to be given if participant fails to recall one or more items in the recall task.

This task should be given to allow the participant a chance to recognize items that he or she could not recall. If the participant recalls the name and address correctly, this test is not needed and the participant scores 5. However, many participants will recall only parts. Start by ticking the correctly remembered items on the shaded column (right-hand side) and then tell them "Let me give you some hints. Was the number (or whatever was forgotten or mistaken) x, y or z?" and so on. Every recognized item scores one point. Maximum score is 5. Adding recalled items to those recognized gives the final score for this part of the test.

Example 1b (based on example 1a)

Tester ticks "Orchard Close" on the right-hand side shaded column because participant had recalled that item. The tester should then ask:	Participant's answers:	
- Was it Jerry Barnes, <u>Harry Barnes</u> or Harry Bradford?	Harry Barnes	1
		0
- Was it 37, <u>73</u> or 76?	76	1
- Was it Oakhampton, <u>Kingsbridge</u> or Dartington?	Kingsbridge	0
- Was it <u>Devon</u>, Dorset or Somerset?	Dorset	+1 (Orchard Close)
		Score 3/5

Example 2b (based on example 2a)

Tester ticks "Harry Barnes", "73" and "Devon" on the right-hand side shaded column because participant had recalled those items. The tester should then ask:	Participant's answers:	
- Was it Orchard Place, Oak Close or <u>Orchard Close</u>?	Orchard Close	1
- Was it Oakhampton, <u>Kingsbridge</u> or Dartington?	Kingsbridge	1 + 3 (Harry Barnes, 73, Devon) **Score 5/5**

Example 3b (based on example 3a)

Tester ticks "Devon" on the right-hand side shaded column because participant had recalled that item. The tester should then ask:	Participant's answers:	
- Was it Jerry Barnes, <u>Harry Barnes</u> or Harry Bradford?	Jerry Barnes	0
- Was it 37, <u>73</u> or 76?	37	0
- Was it <u>Orchard Place</u>, Oak Close or Orchard Close?	Orchard Place	0
- Was it Oakhampton, <u>Kingsbridge</u> or Dartington?	Oakhampton	0 +1 (Devon) **Score 1/5**

MMSE — score 0 to 30

The MMSE score can be obtained by adding up the scores in the shaded boxes to the right-hand side of each test.

Normative data

For the original version of the ACE we derived normative data from 127 controls and recommended the use of two cut-offs (<88 + <82) with high sensitivity and high specificity, respectively. We expected that the revised version might perform differently but we were very pleased to find almost identical results when it was administered to 63 normal volunteer subjects along with 178 clinic attenders (142 with dementia). Again a cut-off of 88 produced high

Table 7.1 Sensitivity and specificity of different ACE-R (and the MMSE) cut-off scores for diagnosing dementia, with corresponding positive predictive values (PPV) at different rates of dementia prevalence

ACE-R cut-off	Sensitivity	Specificity	PPV at different prevalence rates			
			5%	10%	20%	40%
88	0.94	0.89	0.31 (1.0)	0.48	0.68	0.85 (1.0)
82	0.84	1.00	1.0 (0.96)	1.0	1.0	1.0 (0.90)

sensitivity (0.94) but lower specificity (0.89) whereas a cut-off of 82 resulted in lower sensitivity (0.84) but great specificity (1.00). In other words, patients with a score <88 are at high risk of having an organic brain disease, but at this high cut-off you will generate false positives. Conversely, at the lower cut-off (<82) you will almost certainly detect all dementia patients but you will miss cases with early Alzheimer's disease (false negatives). Table 7.1 shows the full sensitivity, specificity and positive predictive values (PPV) at different base rates of dementia and Table 7.2 shows cut-off for the various subscores. In order to tackle the 'grey zone' between 88 and 82, we devised likelihood ratios for probability of dementia. Table 7.3 illustrates that as the ACE-R cut-off falls from 88 to 82, the likelihood ratio rate rises progressively from 8.4 to 100, which means that a score of 82 is 100 times more likely to come from a patient with dementia than one without.

One of the aims of the old ACE was to differentiate AD from FTD. After various attempts we produced a ratio score (VLOM ratio) that reflects the relative balance of cognitive dysfunction in these two disorders:

VLOM ratio = [verbal fluency and language]/[orientation and memory].

Using both the old and the revised ACE, a VLOM ratio of >3.2 was found to be optimal in differentiating AD from FTD (74% sensitivity and 85% specificity), whereas a ratio of <2.2 was highly suggestive of FTD (sensitivity 58% and

Table 7.2 Lower limit of normal (cut-off scores) for total ACE-R and subscores according to age, showing control mean minus two standard deviations

Age range (years)	Education (years)	Total ACE-R score	Attention/ orientation	Memory	Fluency	Language	Visuo-spatial
50–59	12.7	86	17	18	9	24	15
60–69	12.9	85	17	19	8	21	14
70–75	12.1	84	16	17	9	22	14

Table 7.3 Likelihood ratios for probability of dementia at various ACE-R cut-off scores

ACE-R score	Likelihood ratio of dementia
88	8.4
87	11.5
86	14.2
85	18.9
84	27.6
83	52.5
82	100

specificity 95%). Scores between 2.2 and 3.2 were poorly predictive of diagnosis. A number of other groups have reported similar findings and that VLOM is a generally useful adjunct to diagnosis.

Additional Material for Particular Cases

Although we consider the ACE-R to be a good general screening instrument, especially in the context of a memory or cognitive disorders clinic, it is often necessary to supplement the instrument with other tasks targeted towards suspected cognitive dysfunction. A full description of cognitive evaluation is presented in Chapter 5. The tasks described below are 'selected highlights' which have been chosen because either the ACE-R is deficient in this domain (e.g. frontal executive function, praxis, face recognition etc.) or further tests are frequently required to clarify the nature of the deficit (e.g. aphasia or agnosia).

Remote memory

To assess remote memory we typically ask patients about recent news events, which should be tailored towards the patient's interests and cultural setting. In the UK the following are helpful in guiding assessment.

- Recent sporting events: Olympic Games, Football World Cup, Cricket series etc.
- Royal family news
- General elections
- Political scandals and resignations
- Disasters: Tsunami, 9/11 Twin Towers, Brighton bombing
- Wars: Iraq, Afghanistan, Gulf war, Falklands etc.

Frontal executive function

As described earlier in this book, it is notoriously difficult to assess executive function at the bedside. The verbal fluency component of the ACE-R is the most sensitive part but it is often necessary to supplement the ACE-R in patients with suspected frontal pathology.

1. Abstraction: proverb interpretation

- 'A rolling stone gathers no moss'
- 'Too many cooks spoil the broth'
- 'Still waters run deep'
- 'A bird in the hand is worth two in the bush'

2. Similarities

In what way are the following the same?

- 'An apple and a banana'
- 'A coat and a dress'
- 'A table and a chair'
- 'A poem and a statue'
- 'Praise and punishment'

3. Go–No-Go

Patient places hand on table and is asked to raise *one finger* in response to a single tap, but to hold still in response to two taps. The examiner taps the undersurface of the table using a random sequence of single and double taps.

4. Motor sequencing

- Luria three-step: demonstrate hand sequence (fist–edge–palm; see p. 125) five times, and then ask subject to repeat sequence.
- Alternating hand movements: demonstrate sequence five times (start position: one hand has fingers etended and the other has clenched fist, then positions alternate; see p. 126), and then get subject to copy.

5. Cognitive estimates test

This very helpful task is described in the Appendix.

Language

1. Speech production

In patients whose principle complaint is difficulty with speech or language and for those in whom the ACE-R reveals such problems, it is important to evaluate language more thoroughly. It is very helpful to ask the patients to describe a complex scene such as that shown in Figure 7.1. Particular note should be made of: speech rate, dysarthria, phonological or semantic errors, word-finding pauses and grammatical errors.

2. Repeat and define

The following is a useful list of multisyllabic words that can be used to test repetition and comprehension. Patients with phonological processing deficits have difficulty with repetition but can convey the meaning when asked to define these words, whereas those with semantic impairments show the opposite pattern: perfect repetition but poor, or absent, understanding often with vague superordinate responses such as "Is it a flower/animal."

- Caterpillar
- Antelope
- Chrysanthemum
- Stethoscope
- Encyclopedia

3. Comprehension of grammar/syntax

This can be tested using an array of three objects (e.g. pen, keys, watch) placed in front of the patient who is then asked to obey a sequence of commands of increasing syntactic complexity.

- 'Put the pen on the watch.'
- 'Touch the watch with the pen.'

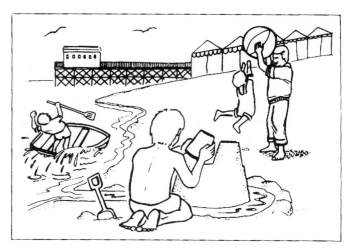

Fig. 7.1 The seaside scene from the Queen Square Screening Test for Cognitive Deficits: an example of a complex interactive scene for use in eliciting spontaneous language. (Reprinted by permission of Professor Elizabeth Warrington.)

Table 7.4 Profile of performance on tests of picture naming, picture description, generation of knowledge and naming from description from the same target names in patients with perceptual, semantic and anomic difficulties

	Perceptual	**Semantic**	**Anomic**
Picture naming	X	X	X
Describe	X	√	√
Knowledge from name	√	X	√
Name from verbal description	√	X	X

X = impaired, √ = intact.

- 'Touch the keys and then the pen.'
- 'Touch the pen before touching the keys.'
- 'Touch the pen but not the keys.'
- 'Put the pen between the watch and the keys.'
- 'You pick up the watch and give me the pen.'

A list of regular, exception and non-words that can be used to screen for types of dyslexia are shown in Table 5.5.

Calculation

Testing basic arithmetic skills should be done in patients with suspected left angular gyrus lesions and is useful in the differentiation of semantic dementia (where calculation is invariably spared) from AD or CBD (in which these abilities are compromised from an early stage). Suggestions are given in Chapter 5.

Praxis

Tests for ideomotor or ideational apraxia are not included in the ACE-R but are important additions in the context of patients with progressive motor syndromes associated with cognitive dysfunction such as PSP and CBD as well as patients with focal left hemisphere pathology.

1. Buccofacial: first to command and then after imitation of examiner

- Blow out a match
- Lick lips
- Cough
- Sip through a straw

2. Limb

(a) Copy of meaningless hand gestures as demonstrated by examiner using right and left hands (see Figure 5.4).

(b) Mime use of objects (combing hair, brushing teeth, using scissors, hammering): first to command then after imitation of examiner.

(c) Symbolic gestures (waving, saluting, beckoning): to command and then after imitation of examiner.

Neglect phenomena

In addition to the drawings in the ACE-R it is useful to screen for suspected neglect using the following tasks.

- Double-headed daisy: ask the patient to copy the figure (Figure 7.2).
- Visual search: using an array of As and Bs unevenly distributed across a sheet of A4 ask the patient to cross out all the As
- Line bisection: ask the patient to mark the half-way point on an array of lines of varying length with a cross (×).

Complex visuo-perceptual abilities and prosopagnosia

Performance on the naming component of the ACE-R should reveal evidence of apperceptual or associative agnosia but the following checklist should help tease apart various causes of object misrecognition and naming (see Table 7.3 for further details).

1. Object agnosia

- Naming of picture/object (note type of error)
- Description of physical appearance of visually presented pictures or objects

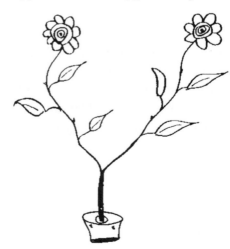

Fig. 7.2 Double-headed daisy in a pot.

- Verbal knowledge about the visually presented stimulus (picture/object)
- Naming from verbal description

2. Prosopagnosia

If a disorder of face recognition is suspected, use pictures of famous people and test the following as described more fully in Chapter 5 (p. 141):

- Face description: ability to describe age, gender, emotion
- Face identification: can they correctly identify the person (e.g. "the Tory woman Prime Minister")
- Face naming: ("Margaret Thatcher")

Chapter 8

Illustrative Cases

This chapter comprises case histories written in short note form that illustrate the method of assessment previously described and the use of the ACE-R. I have not attempted a comprehensive coverage of all cognitive disorders, but have selected a number of recent cases with either important common conditions (such as Alzheimer's disease) or interesting neuropsychological syndromes (such as prosopagnosia). Each case history is followed by a description of the findings on cognitive assessment, a brief differential diagnosis, and a summary of the principal conclusions, indicating whether the services of a neuropsychologist are required or not.

Case 1. Mild Cognitive Impairment (MCI)

Patient: C.G., 62-year-old retired teacher.

History from patient: One to two years' increasing concern over recent memory. Symptoms indicate episodic memory disorder with good attention and preservation of semantic knowledge. No features of depression.

History from family: Confirmed patient's history with some repetitiveness and several incidents of forgetting important events. Preserved activities of daily living.

Past medical history: Nil.

Family history: Mother demented in her 80s.

Physical signs: Nil.

Cognitive assessment

General observations: Appropriate, normal effect.

ACE-R

1. **Orientation and Attention:** Missed only the date, attention intact.

2. **Memory:**

Anterograde: Name and address test: Rapid acquisition of address.

Recall and recognition: Zero recall. Improved with recognition to 3/5.

Retrograde: Normal.

MMSE items: Zero recall of all three words.

3. **Fluency:** Good 'P' words 13 (scaled score = 5) but reduced animal fluency 8 correct with two perseverations (scaled score = 2).

4. **Language:**

Spontaneous speech: Normal.

Naming: All correct (12/12).

Repetition: Normal.

Comprehension: Normal.

Reading: Intact.

Writing: Appropriate sentence with no dysgraphic errors.

5. **Visuo-spatial and perceptual:** Normal.

Mental test scores

	Score	Max
Orientation and Attention	17	18
Memory	15	26
Fluency	7	14
Language	26	26
Visuo-spatial and perceptual	16	16
Overall ACE-R score	**81**	**100**
Overall MMSE score	**26**	**30**

Investigations

MRI scan: Normal.

Differential diagnosis:

- MCI
- Other causes of amnesia (Korsakoff's syndrome etc.)
- Depression

Conclusions: This patient presented with 'organic' symptoms confirmed by a family member. Repetitiveness is particularly concerning. No suggestion of depression. Cognitive screening also points towards significant pathology. Formal neuropsychology is mandatory in this case. An FDG-PET scan revealed marked posterior cingulate cortex hypoperfusion. The patient developed more frank Alzheimer type dementia 3 years later.

Note:
Above 'normal' on MMSE although loss of all three recall points very concerning.
ACE-R detected amnesia and subtle category fluency deficit common in MCI.

Case 2. Early-Stage Alzheimer's Disease

Patient: R.P. 50-year-old farmer's wife.

History from patient: Aware of failing memory, which she has covered up by increasing use of memos and diary, etc. Concentration and general knowledge good. No features of depression (i.e. good energy level and enjoyment of life, no sleep disturbances, etc.). Information about recent personal and public events clearly poor during history taking.

History from family: Two to three years' progressive decline in memory, especially evident for new information, with tendency to repetition. No obvious retrograde memory impairment. Preserved language and practical skills, but some problems managing household accounts and solving problems. Unable to use complicated appliances. No change in personality or behaviour except some loss of motivation.

Past medical history: Nil.

Family history: Mother developed dementia in 50s and died 10 years later, no formal diagnosis was made.

Physical signs: None.

Cognitive assessment

General observations: Normal appropriate behaviour, no mood disturbance.

ACE-R

1. **Orientation and Attention:** Impaired errors on date, day of week and building. Lost one point on serial 7s/WORLD backwards.

2. **Memory:** Impaired.

Anterograde: Name and address test: Normal registration, 7/7 first trial.

Recall and recognition: Very poor delayed recall (0/7) of name and address but improved with recognition: 4 elements correctly identified.

Retrograde: Failed two items.

MMSE items:

3. **Fluency:** Mild reduction, 'P' words 16 but only 13 correct (scaled score = 5), animals 8 (scaled score = 2).

4. **Language:**

Spontaneous speech: Fluent, normal articulation and syntax, no paraphasias.

Naming: 10/12 (hippo for rhinoceros, accordian—don't know).

Repetition: Normal.

Comprehension: Normal.

Reading: Normal.

Writing: Normal spontaneous sentence.

5. **Visuo-spatial and perceptual:** Poor copy of pentagons and cube. Clock poorly organized (3/5). Perceptual tasks (dots and fragmented letters)—normal.

Mental test scores

	Score	Max
Orientation and Attention	14	18
Memory	13	26
Fluency	7	14
Language	23	26
Visuo-spatial and perceptual	11	16
Overall ACE-R score	**68**	**100**
Overall MMSE score	**23**	**30**

Comment: MMSE just below cut-off for 'dementia', lost points for orientation and recall.

Investigations

MRI: Hippocampal atrophy on coronal images (CT not performed, would probably have been normal).

SPECT: Reduced perfusion in bilateral temporo-parietal areas.

Differential diagnosis:

- Early Alzheimer's disease (see p. 38)
- Amnesic syndrome (see p. 15)
- Depressive pseudodementia (see p. 51)

Conclusions: This patient presented with features typical of early Alzheimer's disease, notably a severe amnesic syndrome affecting episodic memory. The remainder of her cognitive function is generally well preserved, but other clues to the diagnosis are the reduced verbal fluency (especially for animals), mild anomia and visuo-spatial deficits. Because of the importance of excluding a depressive pseudodementia a psychiatric opinion should be sought if there is any hint of affective symptoms. Formal neuropsychological assessment is probably optional here if psychiatric features are absent. The early onset and family history raise the possibility of a genetic form of AD (the commonest being a Presenilin I mutation) although the onset is typically even younger.

Note:

- Insight often preserved early in Alzheimer's disease.
- Only just below 'cut-off' on MMSE but clear impairment on ACE-R.
- Formal neuropsychology confirmed more widespread executive–attentional and semantic deficits.
- Genetic testing and counselling is indicated.

Case 3. Moderate Alzheimer's Disease

Patient: A.B., 75-year-old retired handyman.

History from patient: Unaware of deficits, but when challenged admitted memory less good than he would expect.

History from family: Two to three years' insidious decline in memory; now unable to retain any new information. Very repetitive. Grasp of recent events very poor, seems to 'live in the past'. Recently having difficulty with household skills such as cooking, and with hobbies, particularly gardening. Unable to go shopping alone because of difficulty handling money. Speech rather empty, with word-finding difficulty. Preserved social skills and personality but recently apathetic with some irritability. Initially some insight, but now fairly unaware of deficits.

Past medical history: Nil.

Family history: Nil.

Physical signs: None.

Cognitive assessment

General observations: History taking and informal conversation revealed marked amnesia, inattention and language problems.

ACE-R

1. **Orientation and Attention:** Disoriented in time (day, month, date and year) and details of place. Very poor performance on serial 7s/WORLD backwards.

2. **Memory:**

Anterograde: Name and address test: Poor learning, only 4 items even on third trial.

Recall and recognition: No spontaneous recall and recognition impaired (1/5).

Retrograde: Impaired: unable to name any famous figures.

MMSE items: Zero recall of all three words.

3. **Fluency:** Poor, 'P' words 5 (scaled score = 2) and animals 4 (scaled score = 0)

4. **Language:**

Spontaneous speech: Hesitant, some word finding pauses.

Naming: Impaired (6/12), errors included circumlocutions ("thing on a ship" for anchor) and semantic paraphasias (hippo for rhinoceros).

Repetition: Normal for single words but problems with phrases.

Comprehension: Two errors.

Reading: Normal.

Writing: A short but grammatically correct sentence.

5. **Visuo-spatial and perceptual:** Unable to copy pentagons and cube, very poor clock drawing and two errors on dot counting.

Mental test score

	Score	Max
Orientation and Attention	9	18
Memory	5	26
Fluency	2	14
Language	18	26
Visuo-spatial and perceptual	10	16
Overall ACE-R score	**44**	**100**
Overall MMSE score	**16**	**30**

Comment: MMSE well below 'cut-off'; failed most of orientation items, recall of three items, and copy of pentagons.

Investigations

MRI scan: Generalized cortical atrophy with ventricular enlargement.

Differential diagnosis:

- Alzheimer's disease.
- Other causes of dementia.

Conclusions: The cognitive examination revealed very obvious impairment of memory, language, abstract thinking, and constructional abilities typical of moderately advanced dementia of Alzheimer's type. In this instance, formal neuropsychological assessment is unnecessary.

Note:

♦ Despite severity of cognitive deficits, well-preserved social behaviour and personality.

Case 4. Depressive Pseudodementia

Patient: D.A., 67-year-old retired shop assistant.

History from patient: Aware of poor memory and concentration; denied any symptoms of 'depression', but admitted to poor sleep with early-morning waking, low energy, and a lack of interest in the home and family.

History from family: Well until 6 months before, then rapid decline in memory as well as a change in personality, with apathy and disinterest. Poor appetite and sleep pattern. Very complaining and irritable. Preoccupied with negative thoughts.

Past medical history: 'Nervous breakdown' 15 years previously required hospital admission.

Family History: Mother and sister with episodes of depression.

Physical signs: None.

Cognitive assessment

General observations: Poor eye contact, monotonous voice, tendency to give up and produce 'don't know' responses.

ACE-R

1. **Orientation and Attention:** Orientation intact except date but difficulty performing serial 7s/WORLD backwards (score = 2).

2. **Memory:**

Anterograde: Name and address test: Slow acquisition of name and address.

Recall and recognition: Poor recall (2/7) but perfect recognition.

Retrograde: Normal.

MMSE items: Recalled only 1/3 words.

3. **Fluency:** Reduced, 'P' words 8 (scaled score = 4) and animals fluency 10 (scaled score = 3).

4. **Language:**

Spontaneous speech: Normal form and content.

Naming: Perfect.

Repetition: No problems.

Comprehension: Normal.

Reading: Normal.

Writing: Normal.

5. **Visuo-spatial and perceptual:** Normal except slightly poor copy of wire cube.

Mental test scores

	Score	Max
Orientation and Attention	14	18
Memory	20	26
Fluency	7	14
Language	26	26
Visuo-spatial and perceptual	15	16
Overall ACE-R score	**82**	**100**
Overall MMSE score	**23**	**30**

Comment: MMSE lost points on orientation and recall.

Investigations

MRI scan: Normal.

Differential diagnosis:

- Depressive pseudodementia (see p. 51).
- Dementia, especially subcortical type (see p. 36).

Conclusions: Clues to diagnosis in this case are the relatively acute onset; biological features of depression (sleep and appetite); the loss of interest in life; and the family history. Subsequently the patient responded well to treatment with antidepressants. Formal neuropsychological and psychiatric assessment are clearly essential in this case.

Note:

- Just below cut-off on MMSE for 'dementia'.
- Impaired attention and free recall but much better recognition memory.
- Frequent 'don't know' responses.

Case 5. Behavioural Variant Frontotemporal Dementia

Patient: F.M., 64-year-old self-employed builder.

History from patient: Unaware of any problems, and denied symptoms even when directly confronted.

History from family: One to two years of progressive personality change, with lack of motivation, poor judgement, erratic mood swings, lack of empathy over disabled son, and a tendency to crack inappropriate and puerile jokes. Increasing marital disharmony had led to a referral for counselling, since simple 'bedside' mental testing by GP failed to reveal any deficits.

Past medical history: Nil; no excess alcohol intake.

Family History: Mother developed dementia in her late 50s, died in a mental home.

Physical signs: Positive frontal release signs (pout, palmomental, and grasp) only. Sense of smell preserved, discs normal.

Cognitive assessment

General observations: Unconcerned and unaware of reasons for referral. Inappropriate suggestive comments to female staff.

ACE-R

1. **Orientation and Attention:** Perfect in time and place. Two errors in serial subtractions/WORLD backwards (2/5).

2. **Memory:**

Anterograde: Name and address test: Slow acquisition but 7/7 on third trial.

Recall and recognition: Spontaneous recall only 5/7 (mildly impaired) but recognition perfect.

Retrograde: No errors.

MMSE items: Recalled all 3 words.

3. **Fluency:** Impaired, 'P' words 2 (scaled score = 0) and animals 6 (scaled score = 1).

4. **Language:**

Spontaneous speech: Normal form and content.

Naming: No errors.

Repetition: Normal.

Comprehension: Unimpaired.

Reading: Normal.

Writing: An inappropriate ("you're a lovely lady") but otherwise normal sentence.

5. **Visuo-spatial and perceptual:** Mildly disorganized clock drawing.

Additional bedside tests: Unable to interpret proverbs, poor cognitive estimates.

Mental test scores

	Score	Max
Orientation and Attention	16	18
Memory	23	26
Fluency	1	14
Language	26	26
Visuo-spatial and perceptual	14	16
Overall ACE-R score	**80**	**100**
Overall MMSE score	**29**	**30**

Investigations

MRI scan: Mild frontal atrophy with enlargement of anterior part of lateral ventricle.

SPECT: Marked bi-frontal hypoperfusion.

Differential diagnosis: causes of frontal lobe dysfunction

+ Frontotemporal dementia (Pick's disease).
+ Subfrontal meningioma.
+ Sequelae of head injury.
+ Alcohol-related dementia.
+ Huntington's disease.
+ Other basal ganglia degenerative disorders.

Conclusions: This is a typical presentation of progressive frontal dysfunction, which in this case turned out to be due to frontotemporal dementia (Pick's disease). Formal neuropsychological assessment is mandatory, since the cognitive deficits on bedside testing are relatively slight (reduced backwards digit span, poor verbal fluency and abstraction). Probably familial given positive family history.

Note:

+ History from informant most important factor.
+ Near-perfect performance on the MMSE.
+ Borderline overall score on ACE-R but very poor fluency is a tell-tale feature.

Case 6. Progressive Non-Fluent Aphasia (PNFA)

Patient: P.B., 70-year-old retired company executive.

History from patient: Five years' gradual loss of spoken language abilities with speech distortion, leading to difficulties in public speaking and communication with friends and family. Use of telephone impossible. Also problems with written composition.

History from family: Confirmed above history, and that non-linguistic abilities remain unaffected. Still able to play golf, drive, go shopping, and perform DIY jobs. Recently comprehension also becoming impaired.

Family history: Nil.

Past medical history: Nil.

Physical signs: None except mild orobuccal apraxia (unable to cough or click tongue to command).

Cognitive assessment

General observations: Clearly frustrated by speech output difficulty but socially appropriate.

ACE-R

1. **Orientation and Attention:** Perfect.

2. **Memory:**

Anterograde: Name and address test: Impaired repetition due to phonological short-term memory problem, so scored only 3/7 on final trial.

Recall and recognition: Impaired (3) but much better on recognition (4/5).

Retrograde: Normal.

MMSE items: Recalled all 3 words.

3. **Fluency:** Markedly reduced, 'P' words 5 (scaled score = 2) and animals 9 (scaled score = 3).

4. **Language:**

Spontaneous speech: Hesitant and distorted with phonological errors and pauses. Very reduced overall output.

Naming: Mildly impaired (8/12) with phonemic errors.

Repetition: Unable to repeat multisyllabic words but clearly aware of their meaning. Failed both sentence repetition tasks.

Comprehension: Normal single word and conceptual comprehension.

Reading: Unable to read irregular words (surface dyslexic).

Writing: Normal sentence construction and spelling.

5. **Visuo-spatial and perceptual:** Perfect drawing and passed perceptual tests.

Mental test scores

	Score	Max
Orientation and Attention .	18	18
Memory	14	26
Fluency	3	14
Language	15	26
Visuo-spatial and perceptual	16	16
Overall ACE-R score	**66**	**100**
Overall MMSE score	**29**	**30**

Investigations

MRI scan: Mild left peri-sylvian atrophy.

SPECT: Marked left frontotemporal hypoperfusion.

Differential diagnosis:

◆ Progressive non-fluent aphasia (see p. 48).

◆ Stroke, tumours and other space-occupying lesions.

Conclusions: The presentation with a progressive loss of language output and relatively good comprehension is typical of this form of frontotemporal dementia (FTD). The preservation of practical everyday abilities, non-verbal memory and visuo-spatial abilities separates this from aphasia in the context of Alzheimer's or vascular dementia. The nature of the language deficit (i.e. impaired phonology and syntax) is distinct from that found in semantic dementia. Formal neuropsychological evaluation required to confirm normal non-verbal and general intellectual abilities, although mild executive deficits are common in PNFA.

Note:

◆ Bedside assessment might just lead to the mistaken conclusion that memory is equally impaired, since verbal memory is impossible to test.

◆ Digit span reduced because of impaired phonological processing.

◆ Orobuccal apraxia was present.

◆ Slightly older age of onset than other FTD syndrome patients.

Case 7. Semantic Dementia

Patient: J.L., 50-year-old electrician.

History from patient: Twelve-month history of "loss of memory for words"—by which he meant difficulty retrieving names of people, places and things. A great 60s music fan who could no longer remember the names of some of his favourite band members.

History from family: Twelve months or so progressive word-finding difficulty, with more recent impairment of comprehension, especially for more unusual words. For instance, unable to order from menus because of difficulty understanding names of foods. Day-to-day event memory good, and no decline in practical abilities. Increasingly rigid behaviour and fixation about eating certain foods repeatedly.

Past medical history: Nil.

Family history: Nil.

Physical signs: No abnormality detected.

Cognitive assessment

General observations: Fluent conversational language and good autobiography. Socially appropriate.

ACE-R

1. **Orientation and Attention:** Orientation perfect, attention no errors.

2. **Memory:**

Anterograde: Name and address test: Fast learning, 7/7 by third trial.

Recall and recognition: Very poor recall (1/7) but better recognition (4/5).

Retrograde: Unable to name 2 out of 4 famous people.

MMSE items: Recalled only 1/3 words.

3. **Fluency:** Impaired, 'P' words 10 (scaled score = 4) and animals 7 (scaled score = 2).

4. **Language:**

Spontaneous speech: Fluent with normal syntax and phonology but some word finding difficulty and use of substitutions ("thingee").

Naming: Impaired (6/12) with marked familiarity effect (i.e. able to name watch and pen but not camel, anchor, harp, barrel, accordion, crocodile).

Repetition: No errors but unable to define the meaning of any of the words.

Comprehension: Impaired (e.g. "nautical, what's that?").

Reading: Surface dyslexia (regularized soot, pint and dough).

Writing: Normal.

5. **Visuo-spatial and perceptual:** Perfect performance.

Mental test scores

	Score	Max
Orientation and Attention	18	18
Memory	16	26
Fluency	6	14
Language	16	26
Visuo-spatial and perceptual	16	16
Overall ACE-R score	72	100
Overall MMSE score	28	30

Investigations

MRI scan: Left anterior temporal lobe atrophy.

SPECT: Marked asymmetrical temporal hypoperfusion.

Differential diagnosis: Temporal lobe dysfunction secondary to:

- Frontotemporal dementia.
- Alzheimer's disease.
- Post-traumatic temporal lobe damage.
- Herpes simplex encephalitis.

Conclusions: The impairment in naming, verbal fluency, word comprehension and face recognition is secondary to a breakdown in semantic memory, which in this case was due to progressive focal atrophy of the temporal lobes, better known as semantic dementia. Semantic memory impairment also occurs in moderate stages of AD, when episodic memory loss is marked and visuo-spatial deficits are apparent.

Note:

- Above 'cut-off' for dementia on MMSE, despite profound semantic memory impairment.
- Surface dyslexia is a consistent finding in semantic dementia.
- Excellent orientation/attention and visuo-spatial skills.
- Poor verbal memory could lead to mistaken label of AD.
- Early behavioural changes typical of semantic dementia.

Case 8. Progressive Prosopagnosia and Personality Change (right temporal variant of frontotemporal dementia)

Patient: S.E., 60-year-old retired railway-worker.

History from patient: Three years' history of progressive difficulty recognizing people, initially distant friends, more recently even fairly close friends.

History from family: Confirms above, and that his day-to-day (episodic) memory is very good. Also increasingly rigid and cold. Loss of libido and strange preoccupations with religious themes.

Past medical history: Nil.

Family history: Nil.

Physical signs: Nil.

Cognitive assessment

General observations: Very talkative, strange flat affect, difficulty turn taking in conversation.

ACE-R

1. **Orientation and Attention:** Orientation normal for time and place. Attention normal.

2. **Memory:**

Anterograde: Name and address test: Able to learn within 3 trials.

Recall and recognition: Reduced (4/7) but improved on forced choice recognition (4/5).

Retrograde: Only able to name current Prime Minister (1/4).

MMSE items: Recalled all 3 words.

3. **Fluency:** Mildly reduced, 'P' words 13 (scaled score = 5) and animals 10 (scaled score = 3).

4. **Language:**

Spontaneous speech: Normal form and content.

Naming: Within normal limits (11/12).

Repetition: Normal for words and phrases.

Comprehension: Failed two questions (2/4).

Reading: Normal.

Writing: Normal.

5. **Visuo-spatial and perceptual:** Normal drawing and perceptual abilities.

Additional bedside tests: Unable to recognize or name very famous faces (Princess Diana) but also unable to provide information when given the name indicating a cross-modal semantic loss as opposed to the face-specific loss in prosopagnosia after a right temporo-occipital stroke.

Mental test scores

	Score	Max
Orientation and Attention	18	18
Memory	20	26
Fluency	8	14
Language	22	26
Visuo-spatial and perceptual	15	16
Overall ACE-R score	**83**	**100**
Overall MMSE score	**30**	**30**

Investigations

MRI scan: Marked atrophy of anterior right temporal lobe.

FDG-PET: Confirmed bi-temporal hypometabolism (right > left).

Differential diagnosis: Causes of prosopagnosia (see p. 89):

- Right temporal variant of frontotemporal dementia.
- *Herpes simplex* virus encephalitis.
- Posterior cerebral artery territory stroke.
- Carbon monoxide poisoning.

Conclusions: This man's complaint of difficulty in face recognition (prosopagnosia) suggests right temporal lobe dysfunction. Bedside testing points to a loss of semantic memory underlying the face recognition deficit. Formal neuropsychological assessment is clearly important to clarify the deficits and in this case confirmed non-verbal memory deficits plus an agnosia for people and buildings. Also displayed the characteristic changes in social conduct and affect seen in this syndrome.

Note:

- Right temporal lobe function is difficult to assess at the bedside.
- Normal constructional abilities (which depend on parietal lobe function), despite severe prosopagnosia.
- Right temporal lobe damage is associated with personality changes.

Case 9. Corticobasal Degeneration

Patient: C.S., 60-year-old hairdresser.

History of patient: Twelve months' clumsiness, difficulty manipulating scissors and doing other fine hand tasks. Problems writing and spelling. Slight hesitancy of speech and mild slowing of gait. No falls.

History from family: Confirmed patient's history, in addition some "mental slowing", less able to cope with complex situations.

Past medical history: Nil, particularly no vascular risk factor.

Family history: Nil.

Physical signs: Mildly hypomimic, increased tone asymmetric (right > left) with rigidity and cog-wheeling. Bilateral grasping and positive pout response. Marked apraxia (see below). Gait slowed for age with reduced right arm swing.

Cognitive assessment

General observations: Early speech output disorder, normal affect and socially appropriate.

ACE-R

1. **Orientation and Attention:** Normal for time, one error on place.

2. **Memory:**

Anterograde: Name and address test: Impaired learning (5/7 on third trial).

Recall and recognition: Reduced recall (3/7) improved with multiple choice (3/5).

Retrograde: Two errors.

MMSE items: Zero recall of all three words.

3. **Fluency:** Reduced, 'P' words 6 (scaled score = 3) and animals 8 (scaled score = 1).

4. **Language:**

Spontaneous speech: Laboured, hypophonic with word-finding pauses.

Naming: Mildly impaired (8/10).

Repetition: Unable to repeat multisyllabic words or phrases.

Comprehension: Normal.

Reading: Normal.

Writing: Able to write sentence but letters poorly formed and spelling errors.

5. **Visuo-spatial and perceptual:** Very impaired, unable to copy pentagons or cube. Clock face poorly organized (3/5). Also poor on letter identification and dot counting.

Additional bedside tests: Markedly apraxic, unable to copy meaningless gestures especially with right hand. Better at meaningful gestures and improved with imitation (ideomotor). Also early orobuccal apraxia. No overt alien-hand phenomena but uncontrollable tendency to approach the examiner's hand during testing.

Mental test scores

	Score	Max
Orientation and Attention	16	18
Memory	14	26
Fluency	4	14
Language	21	26
Visuo-spatial and perceptual	7	16
Overall ACE-R score	**62**	**100**
Overall MMSE score	**24**	**30**

Investigations

MRI scan: Mild frontoparietal atrophy (left > right).

SPECT: Marked hypoperfusion bilateral frontal and parietal regions.

Differential diagnosis:

- Corticobasal degeneration.
- Progressive supranuclear palsy.
- Dementia with Lewy bodies.
- Vascular dementia.

Conclusions: The combination of asymmetric parkinsonism, apraxia and cognitive deficits is typical of CBD. Patients can present with prominent non-fluent aphasia and/or personality change (see p. 43). MRI may be fairly unremarkable, progression often rapid.

Note:

- Mixture of extrapyramidal and focal cortical features.
- Constructional difficulties could be partially due to apraxia but also impaired perceptual abilities.
- Problems with writing and mild phonological deficits are typical.
- Copying meaningless gestures typically much worse than meaningful.
- Marked discrepancy between MMSE and ACE-R scores.

Case 10. Progressive Supranuclear Palsy (PSP)

Patient: 75-year-old retired teacher.

History from patient: Two years of unsteady gait with a number of unprovoked falls. General slowing. Difficulty reading and going downstairs.

History from family: Confirmed physical history but in addition increasing apathy and lack of spontaneous conversation. Some forgetfulness. No other personality change.

Past medical history: Nil.

Family history: Nil.

Physical signs: Staring facies with slight head retraction. Restricted eye movements especially in vertical plane but preserved oculocephalic reflexes. Nuchal rigidity. Mild bradykinesia and increase limb tone. Slow gait with very deliberate turning. Mild dysarthria but no other bulbar signs.

Cognitive assessment

General observations: Reduced conversation. Slow to respond to questions.

ACE-R

1. **Orientation and Attention:** Fully orientated but slow on serial 7s with two mistakes.

2. **Memory:**

Anterograde: Name and address test: Slow acquisition but learnt all elements by third trial (7/7).

Recall and recognition: Mildly reduced recall (4/7) but perfect of recognition (5/5).

Retrograde: Normal.

MMSE items: Recalled all 3 words albeit slowly.

3. **Fluency:** Markedly reduced, 'P' words 5 (scaled score = 2) and animals 7 (scaled score = 2).

4. **Language:**

Spontaneous speech: Hypophonic, laconic and adynamic with short, correct sentences.

Naming: All correct (12/12).

Repetition: Able to repeat words, one error on phrases.

Comprehension: Normal.

Reading: Normal.

Writing: Correct but minimalist sentence and small poorly executed writing.

5. **Visuo-spatial and perceptual:** Shaky copies but, no errors on perceptual tasks.

Mental test scores

	Score	Max
Orientation and Attention	18	18
Memory	22	26
Fluency	4	14
Language	24	26
Visuo-spatial and perceptual	16	16
Overall ACE-R score	**84**	**100**
Overall MMSE score	**28**	**30**

Investigations

MRI scan: Normal.

Differential diagnosis:

- PSP.
- Multiple system atrophy.
- Corticobasal degeneration.
- Dementia with Lewy bodies.

Conclusions: The combination of history and eye signs is classic for PSP (see p. 50). Some patients have predominantly cognitive presentations with apathy, dysexecutive symptoms or so-called dynamic aphasia (severely reduced output but no phonological, syntactic semantic deficits).

Note:

- Marked reduced fluency especially 'P' words.

Case 11. Dementia with Lewy Bodies

Patient: H.D., 70-year-old retired postman.

History from patient: Two years of "poor memory" with difficulty concentrating and forgetfulness. Some mood disturbance and restless sleep. Occasional fleeting visual hallucinations—ghostlike figures induced by flickering lights and people in the garden. Some day-to-day variation but no periods of gross confusion.

History from family: Confirmed forgetfulness, marked ageing with mental slowing. Also physically slowed.

Past medical history: Nil.

Family history: Nil.

Physical signs: Mildly hypomimic, some bradykinesa and rigidity but no tremor. Gait slowed. Positive frontal release signs.

Cognitive assessment

General observations: Lucid, mildly parkinsonian speech, some word finding pauses.

ACE-R

1. **Orientation and Attention:** Poorly orientated in time (2/5) and unable to perform serial 7s/WORLD backwards.

2. **Memory:**

Anterograde: Name and address test: Poor acquisition over three trials, final score 5/7.

Recall and recognition: Impaired (2/7) but improved on recognition (4/5).

Retrograde: Normal.

MMSE items: Zero recall of all three words.

3. **Fluency:** Markedly reduced, 'P' words 5 (scaled score = 2) and animals 8 (scaled score = 2).

4. **Language:**

Spontaneous speech: Hypophonic with some pauses.

Naming: Mildly impaired (9/12).

Repetition: Unable to repeat phrases.

Comprehension: Normal.

Reading: Normal.

Writing: Micrographic but grammatically correct.

5. **Visuo-spatial and perceptual:** Markedly impaired. Unable to copy pentagons and poor clock drawing (3/5). Also failed on fragmented letters (2/4).

Mental test scores

	Score	Max
Orientation and Attention	8	18
Memory	17	26
Fluency	4	14
Language	21	26
Visuo-spatial and perceptual	9	16
Overall ACE-R score	**59**	**100**
Overall MMSE score	**22**	**30**

Investigations

CT scan: Revealed mild cerebral atrophy.

SPECT: Marked bi-parietal and occipital hypoperfusion.

Differential diagnosis:

- Dementia with Lewy bodies.
- Vascular dementia.
- Alzheimer's disease.

Conclusions: The combination of mood disturbance with cognitive slowing, forgetfulness (but not the striking amnesia of early AD), fleeting hallucinations, visuo-perceptual disturbance and parkinsonism is classic. Some patients may not show motor signs at presentation. Cognitive assessment typically reveals marked deficits in attention and visuo-spatial/perceptual problems (see p. 50).

Note:

- Gross discrepancy between MMSE and ACE-R.
- Combination of attentional, memory and perceptual deficits.
- Sleep disruption and acting out of dreams during REM (rapid eye movement) phase is very common in dementia with Lewy bodies.

Case 12. Visual Variant of Alzheimer's Disease (posterior cortical atrophy)

Patient: P.G., 70-year-old retired technician.

History from patient: 2 years' "loss of vision" with no ophthalmological cause. Unable to locate objects without mis-reaching. Difficulty driving with several minor accidents. Disorientated in unfamiliar environments. Problems reading. No memory or language complaints.

History from family: Family confirmed symptoms and confirmed absence of memory difficulty. No personality change. Some mood disturbance secondary to visual disabilities.

Past medical history: Nil.

Family History: Nil.

Physical signs: Visual fields full but unable to locate and grasp finger of examiner. Acuity apparently very poor using Snellen chart because of problems locating letters but acuity for small print normal.

Cognitive assessment

General observations: Normal affect and memory of interview.

ACE-R

1. **Orientation and Attention:** Normal.

2. **Memory:**

Anterograde: Name and address test: Good learning.

Recall and recognition: Good recall after delay (5/7).

Retrograde: Normal.

MMSE items: Recalled 2/3 words.

3. **Fluency:** Mildly impaired 'P' words 12 (scaled score = 5) and animals 15 (scaled score = 5).

4. **Language:**

Spontaneous speech: Normal form and content.

Naming: Severe difficulty locating target pictures but able to name most if displayed singly by covering others. Two visual-type naming errors (10/12).

Repetition: Normal.

Comprehension: Normal.

Reading and Writing: Normal.

5. **Visuo-spatial and perceptual:** Markedly impaired, unable to copy pentagons or cube. On clock face located numbers outside of circle. Unable to count dots and two errors on fragmented letters.

Mental test scores

	Score	Max
Orientation and Attention	18	18
Memory	23	26
Fluency	10	14
Language	23	26
Visuo-spatial and perceptual	3	16
Overall ACE-R score	**77**	**100**
Overall MMSE score	**27**	**30**

Investigations

MRI scan: Occipito-parietal atrophy.

SPECT: Marked hypoperfusion of parieto-temporal and occipital cortices.

Differential diagnosis:

◆ Posterior cortical atrophy (visual variant AD).

◆ Corticobasal degeneration.

◆ Dementia with Lewy bodies.

◆ Posterior watershed infarction.

◆ Post-CO (carbon monoxide) poisoning.

◆ Creutzfeldt–Jacob disease (CJD).

Conclusions: The history of gradual onset of Balint's syndrome is very characteristic of PCA (see p. 42). Most patients have consulted opticians and ophthalmologists. Memory is typically well preserved. The absence of apraxia or parkinsonism differentiates this from corticobasal degeneration. CJD may start in this way but is more rapidly progressive. MRI may be normal. Neuropsychological evaluation is required. This patient progressed to a state of severe disability but insight and memory remained intact.

Note:

- ◆ Non-specific visual complaints are typical and initially lead to optician and ophthalmological consultations.
- ◆ Memory is usually well preserved.
- ◆ Patients become very disabled.

Case 13. Huntington's Disease

Patient: B.Y., 50-year-old accountant.

History from patient: Unaware of any cognitive deficits; but admitted to excessive fidgetiness for several years.

History from family: Two years' insidious change in personality, with lack of drive and motivation, originally diagnosed as depression. Problems coping at work and disorganized personal finances. Decline in personal care and appearance. Twitchy facial and hand movements noted about the same time by family members.

Past medical history: Nil.

Family history: Father died in his 40s of pneumonia, spent some time in psychiatric care with 'nervous depression'. Paternal grandmother had jerky movements. No explicit diagnosis of Huntington's disease.

Physical signs: Prominent choreiform movements of face, head, and arms. Unsteady reeling gait, with typical finger-flicking. Unable to maintain tongue protrusion. Frontal release signs (pout, palmo-mentals) present.

Cognitive assessment

General observations: Appeared unconcerned and giggly. Easily distracted.

ACE-R

1. **Orientation and Attention:** Orientation largely intact. Attention very poor, unable to do serial 7s/WORLD backwards

2. **Memory:**

Anterograde: Name and address test: Mildly impaired learning, 6/7 after three trials.

Recall and recognition: Impaired free recall (4/7) but much better recognition (5/5).

Retrograde: Intact.

MMSE items: Recalled only 1/3 words.

3. **Fluency:** Markedly reduced, 'P' words 5 (scaled score = 2) and animals 9 (scaled score = 3).

4. Language:

Spontaneous speech: Dysarthric but no aphasic errors.

Naming: Normal (12/12).

Repetition: Mild dysarthria but no phonological errors when repeating words. Failed phrase repetition.

Comprehension: Normal.

Reading: Normal.

Writing: Normal.

5. Visuo-spatial and perceptual: Impaired copy of pentagons, cube and clock (3/5) but normal on perceptual tests.

Mental test scores

	Score	Max
Orientation and Attention	12	18
Memory	22	26
Fluency	5	14
Language	22	26
Visuo-spatial and perceptual	10	14
Overall ACE-R score	**71**	**100**
Overall MMSE score	**21**	**30**

Investigations

MRI scan: Normal.

Differential diagnosis:

- Huntington's disease (see p. 49).
- Wilson's disease.
- Cerebral vasculitis, especially systematic lupus erythematosus (SLE).
- Other very rare causes of chorea and dementia, such as acanthocytosis, etc.

Conclusions: Although the patient presented with chorea and is unaware of any cognitive deficits, bedside testing shows features suggestive of fronto-striatal dysfunction. Initially the family history was said to be negative, but further investigation revealed 'tell-tale' features of Huntington's disease (i.e. a family history of psychiatric illness and involuntary movement disorder). Formal neuropsychological and clinical genetic referral is essential.

Note:

- Cognitive abnormalities relatively subtle; mild attentional deficit, problems with executive function, borderline memory performance, and poor visuo-spatial ability.

- MMSE again above 'cut-off' for dementia.
- CT or MRI scan may show caudate atrophy, but usually only in more advanced cases.

Case 14. Amnestic Stroke: Bilateral Thalamic Infarction

Patient: P.S., 65-year-old retired garage proprietor.

History from patient: Vague recall of hospital admission, but no insight into persistent memory disorder or change in behaviour. Claims to be on active service in the navy and currently at home on shore leave.

History from family: Six months prior to assessment admitted to hospital in coma after being found in bed by wife, unrousable. Rapidly regained consciousness, but severely confused and disorientated. Complex and persistent confabulatory state; believes that it is wartime and that he is on active service. Virtually no recall of past 40 years. Unable to lay down new memories. Complete lack of motivation and drive; previously very active, now watches TV all day.

Past medical history: Hypertension and smoking. No prior cerebrovascular events. Very modest alcohol intake.

Family history: Nil of note.

Physical signs: Disordered eye movements, with paralysis of voluntary vertical gaze.

Cognitive assessment

General observations: Apathetic, extremely poor memory and tendency to confabulate.

ACE-R

1. **Orientation and Attention:** Severely disorientated in time and place.

2. **Memory:**

Anterograde: Name and address test: Able to register and learn address (7/7).

Recall and recognition: No recall (0/7) and chance recognition performance (0/5).

Retrograde: Failed all items.

MMSE: Unable to recall 3 items from MMSE.

3. **Fluency:** Reduced, 'P' words 7 (scaled score = 3) and animals 10 (scaled score = 3) with perseverations.

4. **Language:**

Spontaneous speech: Rather flat but normal form and content.

Naming: Normal (12/12).

Repetition: No errors.

Comprehension: Normal.

Reading: No deficits.

Writing: No deficits.

5. **Visuo-spatial and perceptual:** Careless reproduction of cube and clock drawing.

   Mental test scores

	Score	Max
Orientation and Attention	10	18
Memory	7	26
Fluency	6	14
Language	25	26
Visuo-spatial and perceptual	14	16
Overall ACE-R score	**62**	**100**
Overall MMSE score	**21**	**30**

Comment: MMSE lost points for orientation, and on recall of three items.

Investigations

MRI: Symmetrical bilateral thalamic infarcts involving dorsomedial nuclear group.

Differential diagnosis:

Acute onset of amnesic syndrome (see p. 15), arising from:

- Strokes, either bilateral thalamic or medial temporal.
- Wernicke–Korsakoff's syndrome (B_1 deficiency), usually associated with alcoholism.
- Anoxic hippocampal damage following cardiac arrest, etc.
- *Herpes simplex* virus encephalitis.
- Closed head injury.

Conclusions: The presentation with coma, evolving into an amnesic state with profound anterograde and retrograde memory deficit, is typical of bilateral thalamic infarction. CT scanning is often normal immediately post-stroke, but a subsequent MRI demonstrated the classic lesion. All the vital memory structures are supplied from the posterior cerebral artery. In a high proportion of normal subjects both medial thalamic areas receive supply from a single penetrating artery. Formal neuropsychological assessment is clearly desirable in this case.

Note:

- ◆ Preservation of short-term (working) memory.
- ◆ Evidence of frontal dysfunction due to secondary frontal deafferentation.
- ◆ Eye movement disorder typical of this syndrome.

Case 15. Transient Epileptic Amnesia (TEA)

Patient: L.C., 65-year-old writer.

History from patient: Presenting with recurrent brief (10–15 min) episodes of "confusion" especially just after waking up. Unable to recall anything about the attacks. Also poor recall of recent family events and holidays. For instance, she had spent several weeks in Crete one year before with her husband, an archaeologist, but has no memory of the trip. Previously diagnosed as "psychogenic".

History from family: Husband described sudden onset of amnesia with repetitive questioning and disorientation. No epileptic features (automatisms). Also confirmed autobiographical amnesia.

Past medical history: Nil.

Family history: Nil.

Physical signs: Normal.

Cognitive assessment

General observations: Completely normal on informal assessment.

ACE-R

1. **Orientation and Attention:** Normal.

2. **Memory:**

Anterograde: Name and address test: Good learning, perfect on third trial.

Recall and recognition: Normal.

Retrograde: All correct.

MMSE items: Recalled all 3 words.

3. **Fluency:** Excellent performance, 'P' words 18 (scaled score = 7) and animals 22 (scaled score = 7).

4. **Language:**

Spontaneous speech: Fluent, non-anomic, normal form.

Naming: Perfect.

Repetition: Normal.

Comprehension: Normal.

Reading: Normal.

Writing: Normal.

5. **Visuo-spatial and perceptual:** No deficits.

Mental test scores

	Score	Max
Orientation and Attention	18	18
Memory	25	26
Fluency	14	14
Language	26	26
Visuo-spatial and perceptual	16	16
Overall ACE-R score	**99**	**100**
Overall MMSE score	**30**	**30**

Investigations

MRI scan: Normal.

Differential diagnosis:

- TEA.
- Transient global amnesia (TGA).

Conclusions: The history is very characteristic of TEA with brief recurrent episodes (see p. 14). Although performance on standard neuropsychological tests of memory is normal they show accelerated loss of new information over weeks plus gaps in their autobiographical memory. The diagnosis should be confirmed by routine and, if necessary, sleep EEG.

Note:

- Recurrence is rare in TGA.
- TEA episodes are brief.
- Patients have accelerated forgetting and autobiographical memory loss.

Neuropsychological Tests

A large number of neuropsychological tests are commercially available. Many more, designed initially by psychologists for their own clinical and/or research purposes, have become fairly widely used, but are not published. In this section, I will describe only a fraction of the tests potentially available. The ones I have chosen to describe are either: (i) tests so commonly used by professional neuropsychologists (for example, the Wechsler Intelligence and Memory Scales) that clinicians interested in cognitive function should be aware of their make-up and scoring, if they are going to interpret neuropsychological reports (these tests are, on the whole, fairly time-consuming, and require training in administration, scoring, and interpretation); or (ii) tests that can be regularly used in the clinic or ward, that do not require special training, and that are relatively quick to administer and score (for example, digit span, story recall, Rey figure copy and recall, letter and category fluency tests, etc.). The tests are arranged in alphabetical order. Normative data are given as means with standard deviations (shown as X ± Y). In the case of those tests that are professionally produced and copyrighted, I have given the name of the publishers. The addresses of the major test publishers are listed at the end of the Appendix.

The Autobiographical Memory Interview (AMI) (Harcourt Assessment Resources, Inc.)

The AMI was designed by Kopelman, Wilson and Baddeley to assess personal remote (retrograde) memory. There are two sections: the personal semantic schedule and the autobiographical incident schedule. In the first section, subjects are asked to recall specified *facts* from each of three epochs: childhood (for example, names of teachers and school), early adult life (for example, name of first employer, date and place of wedding), and recent life (for example holidays, journeys, and hospitalizations). Each of these is scored for detail and accuracy by checking with an informant. The second section assesses remote episodic memory. Subjects are asked to recall three specific *incidents* from each of the same life-periods. Scoring is in terms of the descriptive richness of the incident and its specificity to place. Normative data are available, with cut-offs for probable and definite impairment on both sections. The interview has been used in amnesic and demented patients.

Behavioural Assessment of the Dysexecutive Syndrome (BADS) (Harcourt Assessment Resources, Inc.)

This battery was developed by Barbara Wilson and colleagues to predict and measure everyday problems arising from dysexecutive syndromes. It was hoped that it would overcome deficiencies associated with previous tests by including tasks specifically sensitive to skills involved in problem solving, planning, and organizing behaviours over an extended period of time. Several of the subtests are more ecologically orientated than traditional neuropsychological tests and were designed to mimic everyday situations. The overall test battery takes approximately 40–60 min to administer and comprises the following subtests:

1. *Temporal judgement*. This test uses four questions to assess a subject's ability to estimate how long various everyday events (such as a routine dental appointment) typically last.

2. *Rule shift cards*. This tests the ability to change an established pattern of responding using familiar materials and to shift from one rule to another. In the first part of the test, subjects are asked to say "yes" to a red card and "no" to a black card. In the second part of the test the rule is changed. Subjects are asked to respond "yes" if the card that has just been turned over is the same colour as the previously turned card and "no" if it is a different colour. The measures are the time taken and the number of errors.

3. *Action programme test*. In this test of practical problem solving, a cork has to be extracted from a tall tube; a result can only be achieved by a planned use of various other materials provided.

4. *Key search*. This is a test of strategy formation. Subjects are required to demonstrate how they would search a field for a lost set of keys and their performance is scored according to the use of appropriate strategies.

5. *Zoo map*. This is a test of planning. Subjects are required to show how they would visit a series of designated locations on the map of a zoo. When planning the route certain rules must be obeyed. There are two trials. The aims are identical in both trials but the instructions given vary. Subjects are required to visit six out of 12 possible locations. The first trial consists of a high-demand version of the task in which the planning abilities are rigorously tested. To minimize errors, subjects must plan in advance the order in which the designated locations will be visited. In the second, or low-demand, trial, the subjects are simply required to follow the instructions to produce an error-free performance.

6. *The modified six elements test.* This test is based on earlier work by Shallice and Burgess and involves subjects being given instructions to do three tasks (dictation, arithmetic and picture-naming) each of which has been divided into two parts, called A and B. The subjects are required to attempt at least something from each of the six subtests within the 10 min provided.

Also included within the battery is the Dysexecutive Questionnaire (DEX), a 20-item questionnaire constructed in order to sample a range of problems commonly associated with dysexecutive syndromes such as emotional and personality changes, motivational problems and behavioural changes.

For each test, scores are converted into a profile score with the best being a score of four and the worst zero. Extensive normative data on 216 normal subjects in each of three ability bands based on National Adult Reading Test (NART) scores are provided.

The Behavioural Inattention Test (BIT) (Harcourt Assessment Resources, Inc.)

The BIT was developed as a standardized test for detecting and measuring the severity of visual neglect, primarily in stroke and head-injured patients. It has been extensively validated, and normative data exist. It consists of six conventional tests, of which the most sensitive is the Star Cancellation Test, and nine behavioural tests which use everyday situations to judge visual neglect. Normative data are available, and the battery has now been widely used in stroke patients to assess neglect phenomena.

1. The six conventional tests:
   - Line crossing (Albert's test)
   - Letter cancellation
   - Star cancellation
   - Figure and shape copying
   - Line bisection
   - Representational drawing

2. The nine behavioural tests:
   - Picture scanning
   - Telephone dialling
   - Menu reading
   - Article reading
   - Telling and setting the time
   - Coin sorting

- Address and sentence copying
- Map navigation
- Card sorting

The Boston Naming Test (BNT) (Harcourt Assessment Resources, Inc.)

The BNT consists of 60 line drawings, graded from very familiar, high-frequency items such as bed, tree and pencil through to low-frequency items such as trellis, palette and abacus. Adults start with item 30 and proceed forward unless they make mistakes in the first eight items. Standard stimulus cues (for example, pencil 'used for writing') and phonetic (first-syllable) cues are given if items are unnamed. The test has been widely used in aphasia studies. Fairly extensive normative data are available. There is also a shortened 15-item version of the test.

California Verbal Learning Test (CVLT and CVLT-11) (Harcourt Assessment Resources, Inc.)

The CVLT is designed to assess the use of semantic associations as a strategy for learning words. Each of the 16 words in the CVLT list belongs to one of four categories of shopping list items: for example, list A, Monday's list, contains four names of fruits, four of herbs and spices, four of articles of clothing and four of tools; list B, the Tuesday interference list, also contains the names of fruits and of herbs and spices plus four kinds of fish and four kitchen utensils. Category items are presented in a randomized order with instructions to recall the words in any order, thereby assessing the subject's spontaneous use of semantic associations. CVLT performance is a measure of the interaction between verbal memory and conceptual ability. The procedure is similar to the older Rey Auditory Verbal Learning Test (see p. 236). Following five trials of list A, the interference list B is read to the subject. Two short-delay recalls of list A are obtained. The first of the two recall trials is a "free" recall in which the request for the subject to "tell me all" remembered items from list A is identical to the RAVLT free recall procedure. Immediately following the free recall trial the examiner asks the subject to recall items in each of the four semantic categories ("cued" recall). For subjects who use semantic clustering during the learning, cueing at delayed recall offers little additional benefit. However, subjects who fail to make the semantic associations during the learning trial often benefit from cueing. There is then a long delay recall at 20 min under the same two conditions, "free" and "cued", followed by a recognition trial in which subjects have to recognize items presented from a mixture of the following categories: list items, non-list items from the presented categories, items bearing a phonetic resemblance to the list items and items that one might find in a supermarket but were not included in the lists.

In addition to the acquisition scores for trials 1–5, "free" and "cued" recall of list A for short and long delays, the test also allows a number of other scores to be derived including recall consistency, semantic clustering, perseverations, false positives and intrusions. The CVLT manual provides normative data for 273 males and females in seven age-bands covering ages 17–80 years. The CVLT has been shown to be sensitive to memory problems in early Alzheimer's disease, Parkinson's disease, frontal lobe disorders, multiple sclerosis and a range of other forms of organic brain disease.

Cambridge Neuropsychological Test Automated Battery CANTAB (Cambridge Cognition)

The CANTAB battery was originally developed by Sahakian, Robbins and colleagues in Cambridge. It is administered on a computer screen producing, therefore, both reaction time and error scores. The tests in the battery were derived from findings in non-human primate research in an attempt to develop tasks that were sensitive and specific to focal brain damage. It has been extensively used, particularly in a research setting and more recently in pharmacological studies. There are extensive normative data in more than 2000 subjects covering the age range 4–90 years in four different IQ bands. It now consists of 22 tests as listed below.

1. *The Cambridge gambling task.* This was developed to assess decision-making and risk-taking behaviour outside of a learning context. The subject is presented with a row of 10 boxes across the top of the screen, some of which are red and some of which are blue. At the bottom of the screen are rectangles containing the words red and blue. The subject must guess whether a yellow token is hidden in one of the red or blue boxes at the top of the screen. The subject starts with a number of points displayed on the screen and can select which proportion of these points to gamble, based on his/her confidence.

2. *Choice reaction time.* This is a two-choice reaction time test for stimulus and response uncertainty, with two possible stimuli and two possible outcomes.

3. *The graded naming test* (see p. 230).

4. *Simple reaction time.* This measures simple reaction time through delivery of a known stimulus to a known location. The only uncertainties are with regard to when the stimulus will occur and by having a variable interval between trial response and the onset of the stimulus for the next trial.

5. *Big/little circle*. This is a test of the subject's ability to follow an explicit instructional rule and then to reverse this rule. The subject is presented with a series of pairs of circles, one large and one small. The subject is instructed first to follow the smaller of the two and then after 20 trials to touch the larger.

6. *Delayed matching to sample*. The subject is presented with a complex visual pattern (the sample) and then, after a brief delay, four patterns, between which he/she must choose.

7. *ID/ED shift*. This test is broadly based on the Wisconsin Card Sorting Test (see p. 256) and tests the subject's ability to attend to the specific attributes of a compound stimulus, and then to shift that attention when required. Two artificial dimensions are used, colour-filled shapes and white lines. Two stimuli (one correct, one incorrect) are displayed, initially each with only one dimension, then each with both dimensions. Feedback teaches the subject which stimulus is correct, and after six correct responses the stimulus and/or rules are changed. These shifts are initially intra-dimensional (e.g. colour-filled shapes remain the only relevant dimension), then later extra-dimensional (white lines become the only relevant dimension).

8. *Matching to sample visual search*. This is a speed accuracy trade-off test in which subjects match visual samples. An abstract pattern, composed of four coloured elements is presented in the middle of the screen. After a brief delay, a varying number of similar patterns are shown in a circle around the edge of the screen; only one of these matches the pattern in the centre and the subject must indicate which by touching it.

9. *Motor screening*. This is a screening test administered before the other tests to simply estimate the subject's motor speed.

10. *Paired Associate Learning (PAL)*. The PAL is a form of delayed response procedure, which tests the subject's ability to form visuo-spatial associations. Abstract coloured patterns are displayed in boxes around the edge of the screen, increasing in string length from two up to eight sequences. The individual patterns are then displayed in the centre of the screen and the subject must recall the spatial location in which the pattern occurred. This test has been shown to be exquisitely sensitive to early Alzheimer's disease.

11. *Pattern recognition memory*. Subjects are presented with a series of visual patterns in the centre of the screen that cannot easily be given verbal labels. In the recognition phase, subjects are required to choose between a

pattern they have already seen and a novel pattern. The test patterns are presented in the reverse order to the original order of presentation.

12. *Rapid visual information processing.* This is a test of vigilance or sustained attention with a small working memory component. Digits from 2 to 9 appear in pseudo-random order at the centre of the screen at a rate of 100 digits per minute. Subjects are requested to detect consecutive odd or even sequences of digits and to register response using a press pad.

13. *Line reaction time.* This test has five stages of increasingly complex chains of responses. In each case the subject must react as soon as yellow dots appear on the screen. At some stage it may appear in one of five locations and the subject sometimes responds by using a press pad, sometimes by touching the screen and sometimes by touching both.

14. *Spatial recognition memory.* The subject is presented with white squares that move in sequence to five places on the screen. In the recognition phase, the subject sees a series of five pairs of squares, one of which is in the place previously seen in the presentation phase.

15. *Spatial span.* This is a test of spatial memory span. White squares are shown, some of which momentarily change in colour in a variable sequence. The subject must touch each of the boxes in the same order as they were originally coloured by the computer.

16. *Spatial working memory.* This test is designed to assess spatial working memory and strategy performance. The aim of the test is that the subject should find a blue token in each of the boxes displayed and use them to fill up an empty column on the right-hand side of the screen, while not returning to boxes where a blue token has previously been found. The colour and position of the boxes used are changed from trial to trial to discourage the use of stereotyped search strategies.

17. *Stockings of Cambridge.* This task is based upon the famous "Towers of London" test. The subject is shown two displays containing three coloured balls, presented so they can be perceived as a stack of coloured balls in stockings. In each trial, the subject must move the balls from the lower display to copy the pattern shown in the upper display. The number of moves required reflects the subject's planning ability.

18. *Affective go/no-go.* This new inclusion in the battery tests affective cognitive functions thought to be related to ventral and medial–prefrontal cortical regions. The test consists of blocks, each of which presents a series of words from two out of three different affective categories: positive (e.g. joyful), negative (e.g. hopeless) and neutral (e.g. element). The subject

is given a target category and asked to press the keypad when they see words matching to this category, giving latency and correct/incorrect scores.

19. *Verbal recognition memory.* This assesses immediate and delayed memory for verbal information under free recall and forced-choice recognition conditions. In this task, subjects are shown 12 words and then asked first to reproduce as many of the words as possible following presentation, then to recognize words they have seen from a list of 24 containing the original 12 words and 12 distracters. After a delay of 20 min they are asked to recognize the words they saw before from another list of 24 containing the original 12 words and 12 new distracters.

20. *Information Sampling Task.* This assesses impulsivity and decision-making. In this task, the subject is presented with a 5×5 array of grey boxes on the screen, and two larger coloured panels below these boxes. The subject is instructed that they are playing a game for points, which they can win by making a correct decision about which colour is in the majority under the grey boxes. They must touch the grey boxes one at a time, which open up to reveal one of the two colours shown at the bottom of the screen. Once a box has been touched, it remains open. When the subject has made their decision about which colour is in the majority, they must touch the panel of that colour at the bottom of the screen to indicate their choice. After the subject has indicated their choice, all the remaining grey boxes on the screen reveal their colours and a message is displayed to inform the subject whether or not they were correct. The colours change from trial to trial.

There are two conditions – the fixed win condition, in which the subject is awarded 100 points for a correct decision regardless of the number of boxes opened, and the decreasing win condition, in which the number of points that can be won for a correct decision starts at 250 and decreases by 10 points for every box touched. In either condition an incorrect decision costs 100 points.

21. One-touch Stockings of Cambridge. This is a variant of the Stockings of Cambridge task (see page 221). The subject is first required to solve introductory problems in the same way as for Stockings of Cambridge, by moving the balls from the lower display to copy the pattern shown in the upper display, and is then presented with problems where they must not move the balls on the screen but must instead work out the number of moves required to solve each problem, then touch a numbered box at the bottom of the screen to indicate their response.

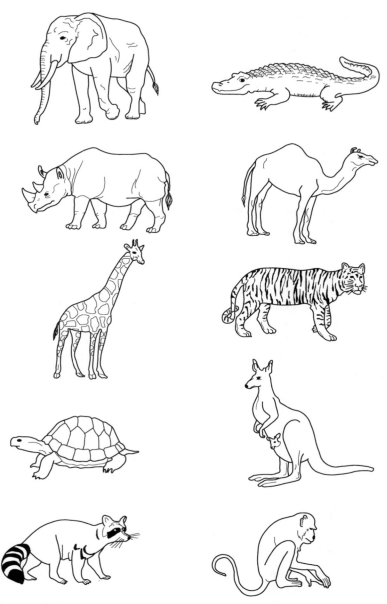

Fig. A1 Word–picture matching subtest from the Cambridge Semantic Battery. (Adapted with permission of Cambridge Cognition.)

22. Stop Signal Task. This gives a measure of an individual's ability to inhibit a prepotent response. This task consists of two parts: in the first part, the subject is introduced to the press pad, and told to press the left hand button when they see a left-pointing arrow, and the right hand button when they see a right-pointing arrow. There is one block of 16 trials for the subject to practice this.

In the second part, the subject is told to continue pressing the buttons on the press pad when they see the arrows, as before, but, if they hear an auditory signal (a beep), they should withhold their response and not press the button.

Cambridge Semantic Memory Test Battery (available from the author)

This battery was developed in the early 1990s to assess the status of semantic memory in patients with neurodegenerative disorders and has proven extremely valuable over the years. It has not been formally published. The battery employs a consistent set of stimulus items and is designed to assess input to, and output from, a putative central semantic store of knowledge via different sensory modalities. The original version of the battery was based on 48 items chosen to represent three categories of natural kinds (animals, sea creatures and birds) and three categories of artefacts (household items, vehicles and musical instruments) which were matched for prototypicality and word frequency. The subsequent version was modified and extended to increase the number of items to 64 with better matching based upon familiarity and age of acquisition. In the newer version of the battery the natural kinds comprise domestic animals (for the UK), foreign animals, fruit and birds while the artefacts are large household items, small household items, vehicles and tools. The following subtests comprise the battery.

1. Category fluency for each of the eight categories with 1 min allowed per category.

2. Naming of all 64 line drawings without cueing.

3. Naming in response to a verbal description such as "the aircraft that can take off and land vertically, and hovers".

4. Word-picture matching (category comprehension subtest) in response to the spoken word using within-category arrays (see Figure A1). Subjects are presented with picture arrays comprising eight items from the same category (six pictures of items included in the battery and two others).

5. Picture and word sorting at different levels within the semantic hierarchy. At level one, subjects are asked to sort between living and man-made things. At level two, the sorting is based on broad categories such as animals vs fruit and at the lowest level three judgements are made according to specific attributes.

6. Generation of verbal definitions. Subjects are asked to provide definitions in as much detail as possible as if describing the item to someone who has never seen one before. Two practice items are given with feedback on these items only. Responses are scored according to their richness and detail according to a standardized proforma.

7. The Camel and Cactus Test. This was developed to be a direct parallel to the Pyramids and Palm Trees test based upon the 64 items from the semantic battery. Subjects have to choose between one of four possible pictures that best goes with the target picture.

Our standard assessment battery contains category fluency, naming, word–picture matching and the Camel and Cactus Test for pictures. The other tests have been used in various research projects. Limited normative data are available. This is clearly a research test battery rather than one applicable for general clinical usage. It is extremely valuable in the assessment of patients with suspected semantic dementia and other rarer disorders involving semantic memory.

Cognitive Estimates Test

In this task, devised by Shallice and Evans, patients are asked to make estimates such as "What is the largest object normally found in the house?" and "How fast do racehorses gallop?" The questions cannot be answered directly from general knowledge. They require novel reasoning, and a comparison with information in the individual's store of knowledge. Patients with frontal lobe disorders give bizarre answers, when are often not easily modified by asking the patients to reconsider their answers. The specificity and sensitivity of the test have not been well studied, but since there are no good alternative tests it remains clinically useful. A modification of the original test (which contained 15 questions) is given below. The test is introduced by saying "I'd like you to make the best guess you can in answer to these questions. Almost certainly you won't know the correct answer, but just make your best guess." Each answer is scored for unusualness or extremeness. Answers in the correct range score 0. Some responses have to be interpolated, since the scoring system given below cannot cover all possibilities.

Box A1 Cognitive Estimates Test

Questions and error scores   *Correct range*

1. What is the height of the London BT Tower?   100–800 feet

> 1500	3	< 60	3
= 1500	2	= 60	2
> 800	1	< 100	1

2. How fast do racehorses gallop?   15–40 m.p.h.

> 50	3	< 9	3
= 50	2	< 15	2
> 40	1		

3. What is the best-paid job in Britain today?   Queen/film or

manual worker	3
blue-collar worker	2
professionals	1

pop-star/sportsman/
Prime Minister, etc.

4. What is the age of the oldest person in   104–113 years
    Britain today?

> 115	3	< 103	3
= 115	2	= 103	1
= 114	1		

5. What is the length of an average man's spine?   1'7"–3'11"

> 5'0"	3	< 1'6"	3
> 4'0"	2	= 1'6"	2
= 4'0"	1		

6. How tall is the average English woman?   5'3"–5'8"

> 6'0"	3	< 5'2"	3
= 5'11", 6'0"	2	= 5'2"	1
= 5'11", 5'10"	1		

7. What is the population of Britain?   20–60 million

> 1000 million	3	< 2 million	3
> 500 million	2	< 5 million	2
= 500 million	1	< 20 million	1

Box A1 Cognitive Estimates Test (continued)

8. How heavy is a full pint of milk?   1–3 lb (17–43 oz)

> 3 lb	3	< 1 lb	3
= 3 lb	1	= 1 lb	1

9. What is the largest object normally found   Bed, bath, etc.
   in a house?

< carpet	3
carpet	2
piano, cupboard, sofa	1

10. How many camels are there in Holland?   1–50

very large number	3
none	1

Controls obtain mean error score of 4.0 (± 2.0)

Delis–Kaplan Executive Function System (D-KEFS) (Harcourt Assessment Resources, Inc.)

The D-KEFS is a set of nine tests, each intended to stand alone. The tests were selected to be sensitive to types of executive impairment seen in patients with brain disorders. The subtests comprise trail making, verbal fluency (letter, category and design fluency), a version of the colour–word interference or Stroop test (see p. 242), a sorting test, the 20 questions test, a Tower of London type test, and a proverbs test. It has the advantage that the tests were all normed on 1750 participants aged 8–89 years and alternative forms are available for some of the subtests. As yet, limited data are available from patient populations.

Digit Span

Digit span is a widely used test of auditory verbal short-term (working) memory. What it measures is more closely related to the efficacy of phonological and attentional processes than to what is commonly thought of as memory (see p. 8). Variations of the task are included in the Wechsler Memory and Intelligence Scales, in which the administration and scoring methods used to obtain raw scores and age-scaled scores differ slightly.

In clinical practice the following method is appropriate for determining forward and reverse digit span. For digits forwards, subjects are asked to repeat back progressively lengthening strings of digits in the same order as they are given by the examiner. A practice trial of 2 digits is given, followed by the progressively lengthening strings as shown below. It is important that the digits are read at one per second without clustering. Two different series are given for each string-length. If the subject passes the first or the second, the next length is given. If both are failed, the test is discontinued. The score is the longest series correctly repeated. For reverse digit span, exactly the same method is used, except that the subject is asked to repeat back the digits in reverse order. Again a trial of 2 digits is given initially (see Box A2).

The normal range for digits forwards is 6 ± 1. Even this simple test is affected by age and educational level. Spans of 6 or better are within normal limits; a span of 5 may be marginal or normal, depending on the age and education of the subject; a span of 4 is definitely borderline or impaired; and a span of 3 is always defective. Reverse digit span is 5 ± 1. Hence a reverse span of 3 is borderline or defective, depending upon age and education, and 2 is always defective. In any individual, the difference between forward and backward digit span should not exceed 2.

Box A2 Digit span

Digits forwards		Digits backwards	
9—7	2		
4—1	2		
4—8—1	3	6—2	2
6—3—2	3	1—9	2
6—4—3—9	4	2—8—3	3
7—2—8—6	4	4—1—5	3
4—2—7—3—1	5	3—2—7—9	4
7—5—8—3—6	5	4—9—6—8	4
6—1—9—4—7—3	6	1—5—2—8—6	5
3—9—2—4—8—7	6	6—1—8—4—3	5
5—9—1—7—4—2—3	7	5—3—9—4—1—8	6
4—1—7—9—3—8—6	7	7—2—4—8—5—6	6
5—8—1—9—2—6—4—7	8	8—1—2—9—3—6—5	7
3—8—2—9—5—1—7—4	8	4—7—3—9—1—2—8	7
Forward score	—	Backward score	—

Digit span is generally vulnerable to focal left hemisphere and frontal lesions. Disorders of attention (for example, delirium or acute confusional states) cause severe reduction, especially in reverse digit span. In Alzheimer's disease, digit span is well maintained initially; but it is reduced in subjects with sub-cortical dementias.

Doors and People Test (Harcourt Assessment Resources, Inc.)

This test was designed by Alan Baddeley and colleagues to provide comparable measures of visual and verbal memory tested by recall and recognition. It produces scores in normal subjects that avoid floor and ceiling effects and incorporates learning and forgetting measures. It takes approximately 20 min to administer and comprises of four subtests: two visual and two verbal.

1. *Visual recognition, the doors test.* The stimuli in this test comprise coloured photographs of doors. There are 27 target doors and 81 distracters. The target doors are mounted singly and for the recognition set each target is presented with three distracters in a 2 × 2 matrix. Three of the items are for practice and the remaining targets are in two sets of 12, an easy set (A) and a harder set (B).

2. *Visual recall, the shapes test.* The stimuli for this test are four line drawings of crosses. There is an immediate and a delayed recall component.

3. *Verbal recognition, the names test.* The test stimuli are forename–surname pairs. As with the doors test, there are 27 target names and 81 distracters. The target names are mounted singly on white cards. For the recognition test, targets are presented with three distracters. There are two subtests, 'A' comprising of easy names and 'B' more difficult names.

4. *Verbal recall, the people test.* The stimuli comprise forename–surname pairs. Each name is paired with an occupation and presented to the subject as a caption to a coloured photograph, a clean-shaven, bespectacled, 40-year-old has the label Jim Green, Doctor.

Normative data are available on 239 subjects stratified in four age-bands from between 16 and 79 years. In addition to raw and age-scaled scores for the four individual tests it is possible to derive composite visual and verbal recall and recognition scores as well as a total memory score and visual–verbal recall discrepancy scores.

The test is used to evaluate patients with suspected episodic memory deficits and is sensitive to early Alzheimer's disease and to the effects of temporal lobectomy.

The Graded Naming Test (GNT) (Cambridge Cognition)

This was designed by McKenna and Warrington to be a stringent test of naming ability, sensitive to mild degrees of anomia. It consists of 30 line drawings, ranging from low frequency (for example kangaroo, scarecrow, and buoy) to very low frequency (for example centaur, mitre, and retort). Some examples are shown below (Figure A2). Expected scores, based on the WAIS Vocabulary and reading ability, can be calculated. Detailed normative data are available.

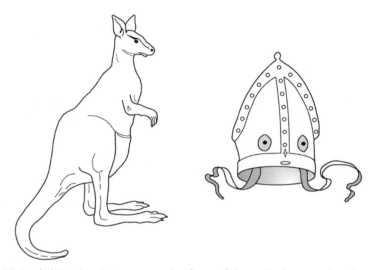

Fig. A2 Graded Naming Test: an example of one of the easier (kangaroo) and one of the harder (mitre) items from the test. (Reprinted by permission of Cambridge Cognition.)

Hayling and Brixton Test (Harcourt Assessment Resources, Inc.)

These tests were developed by Burgess and Shallice to assess aspects of frontal executive function: the ability to inhibit a prepotent response (Hayling) and concept formation (Brixton). The Hayling sentence completion test consists of two sections, each comprising 15 sentences which are missing the last word, such as "The old house will be torn . . . ." The examiner reads aloud each sentence to the subject who is required to make a verbal response. In section one, the subject is asked to complete the sentence sensibly as quickly as possible. In section two, the subject is asked to give a word that is *unconnected* to the sentence in every way. For example "The captain wanted to stay with the sinking . . . light bulb." This test is based on the ability of normal subjects to inhibit a prepotent response.

The test yields three measures. The first is the sum of the response latencies in section one. Section two yields two measures of response suppression comprising the time taken and the number of errors. Each response in section two is classified as falling into one of three categories: the first is where the word produced is completely unconnected to the sentence, as required (this scores zero error points); the second type of response is one which is somewhat connected in meaning to the sentence but not a direct sentence completion; the third type of response is where the subject completes the sentence in an entirely plausible fashion. Control data are available for 120 healthy volunteers. It has been shown to be sensitive to unilateral and bilateral frontal lobe damage as a result of structural brain injury and has been applied to patients with frontotemporal dementia.

The Brixton test measures the ability to detect rules in sequences of stimuli and concept formation. It comprises 56 nearly identical cards printed with 10 (2 rows of 5 each) circles, one of which is coloured while the others are white; the position of each succeeding coloured circle is determined by one of nine rules based on the position of the coloured circles on preceding cards (see Figure A3). On being told that the coloured circle "moves around according to various patterns that come and go without warning", the subject is asked to state the expected position of the coloured circle on the next card. For the first and simplest rule the coloured circle advances one position clockwise on successive cards and a later rule has the circle alternating from place 5 to place 10. Limited normative data are available but frontal patients are reported to make more errors and to respond in a random and unconstrained fashion.

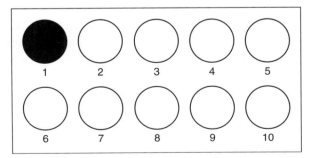

Fig. A3 Example from the Brixton Spatial Anticipation Test. Hayling and Brixton Tests. Copyright © 1997 by Paul W. Burgess and Tim Shallice. Reproduced with permission of Harcourt Assessment Inc.

Judgement of Line Orientation Test (JLO) (NFER—Nelson)

This task, designed by Benton and colleagues, examines the ability to judge and match angular relationships. The subject views pairs of lines with various orientations, and is required to estimate their angulation with reference to a display of 11 numbered lines spanning 180 degrees, which are viewed simultaneously with the target lines (see Figure A4). The test consists of 30 trials of increasing difficulty. It is quick and easy to administer, and comes with several parallel forms. Reasonable normative data are available. The test is sensitive to focal right parietal lesions. It is also failed consistently by patients with Alzheimer's disease beyond the earliest stages.

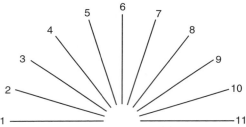

Fig. A4 Judgement of Line Orientation Test. Reproduced with special permission of the Publisher, Psychological Assessment Resources, Inc., from the Judgement of Line Orientation by Authur L. Benton. © 1983 by PAR, Inc.

The National Adult Reading Test: Second Edition (NART)

The NART was developed by Nelson and O'Connell as a quick and simple test to estimate premorbid IQ in patients suspected of suffering from intellectual deterioration. The 50 words constituting the NART are all irregular (DEBT, AISLE, DEPOT, THYME, BOUQUET, PLACEBO, etc.), in that they cannot be pronounced correctly by applying the usual rules of spelling-to-sound correspondence. For example, the word NAIVE would be pronounced 'nave' if one were to decode it phonetically. The principles underlying the test are: (i) that the pronunciation of irregular words depends upon pre-existent familiarity with their meaning; and (ii) that reading is a highly overlearnt skill, which is maintained at a high level despite deterioration in other areas of intellectual functioning.

The 50 words of the test are graded in frequency of occurrence in the English language; the initial items (ACHE, DEBT, PSALM) are familiar to the average adult, while the last words (LABILE, SYNCOPE, PRELATE) are beyond most people's vocabulary. On the basis of the number of errors produced, a premorbid IQ can be estimated in the range 90–128. For subjects below this range the Schonell Graded Word Reading Test should be used. A parallel version, the American National Reading Test (ANART) was developed for an ethnically diverse US population.

While the test remains a valid instrument for estimating premorbid IQ levels in patients with mild dementia, recent research suggests that NART performance declines in moderate Alzheimer's disease. Patients in whom there is a breakdown of the whole-word (lexical) reading route, surface dyslexics, are particularly impaired at reading irregularly spelt words. Their premorbid IQ should be assessed using other measures, such as Raven's Matrices, rather than the NART.

Paced Auditory Serial Addition Test (PASAT) (Brain Metric Software)

This sensitive test requires the subject to add 60 pairs of randomized digits so that each is added to the digit immediately preceding it. For example, if the examiner reads the numbers "2–8–6–1–9", the subject correct response beginning as soon as the examiner reads 8 are "10–14–7–10". The digits are presented at four rates of speed each differing by 0.4 s and ranging from one every 1.2 s to one every 2.4 s. The performance can be evaluated in terms of the percentage of correct responses or the mean score for all trials. It is a difficult task and performance declines with age. It has been found to be particularly sensitive to brain trauma following head injury interpreted as reflecting abnormally slowed information processing. The test is experienced as stressful and is typically only given to high-ability subjects to detect subtle attentional deficits.

Pyramids and Palm Trees Test (Harcourt Assessment Resources, Inc.)

This test, devised by Howard and Patterson, assesses a person's ability to access detailed semantic knowledge from words and from pictures. It can be given in several formats (picture–picture, word–word, picture–word); but the picture–picture-matching version is perhaps the most useful, since it assesses non-verbal semantic knowledge. There are 52 items in the test. The subject is presented with three pictures on a single card (see Figure A5), the target picture is displayed at the top. The subject has to decide which of the two lower pictures is most closely associated with the target. Examples include an Egyptian pyramid with a fir tree and a palm tree (hence the name of the test); spectacles with eye and ear; and saddle with goat and horse. The test remains

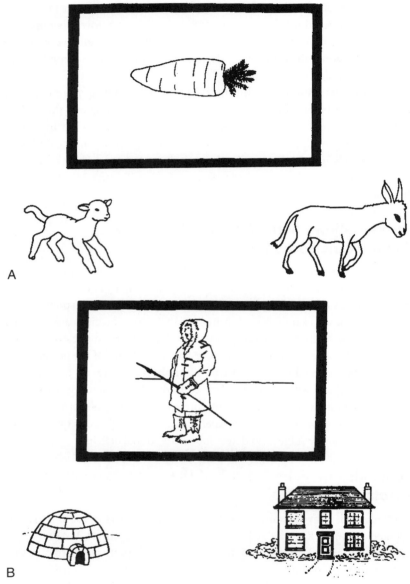

Fig. A5 Pyramids and Palm Trees Test: A and B are two examples from the test. Copyright © 1992 by David Howard and Karalyn Patterson. Reproduced with permission of Harcourt Assessment, Inc.

largely a research tool, but its usage is likely to increase, since there are few good alternatives. Normative data are, at present, rather limited. Normal controls make three or fewer errors on the picture–picture-matching version; patients with semantic memory impairment make considerably more.

Raven's Progressive and Coloured Progressive Matrices (Harcourt Assessment Resources, Inc.)

Raven's Progressive Matrices (RPM) was developed as a 'culture-fair' test of general intellectual inability, although it has subsequently emerged that educational level has a major effect on normal subjects' performance. It consists of 60 visually based problem-solving tests arranged in blocks of increasing complexity. The initial test items require only pattern matching; the subject is faced with a large design, part of which is missing; below are six different small pattern-samples, one of which the subject chooses to complete the larger design above. As the test progresses, the items become more complex, requiring reasoning by analogy rather than simple pattern matching (see Figure A6). The test is simple to administer, but takes 45 min or so to complete. Detailed normative data with percentile scores are available for ages 8–65 years.

Raven's Coloured Progressive Matrices (RCPM) provide a simplified 36-item format, with norms for children and adults aged over 65 years. It has also been used in neuropsychological practice. A greater proportion of the test items are of the pattern-matching type than in the RPM.

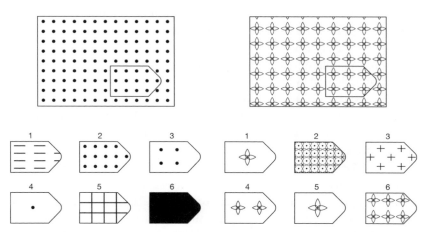

Fig. A6 Raven's Standard Progressive Matrices: example of two of the easier pattern-matching items from the test. Copyright © by Harcourt Assessment Resources, Inc. Reproduced with permission.

Both tests are sensitive to brain damage in fairly widely distributed areas, since normal performance depends upon intact visuo-perceptual, attentional and problem-solving skills. In the absence of visuo-perceptual deficits it is a reasonable test of frontal lobe function.

Recognition Memory Test (RMT) (Harcourt Assessment Resources, Inc.)

This easy-to-administer test of word and face recognition memory was devised by Warrington. In the face memory part, the subject is shown 50 black-and-white photographs of unfamiliar male faces. The examiner asks the subject to attend to each for 3 s and to say whether the faces are pleasant or not. After viewing all 50 faces, subjects are then shown pairs of faces, one of which was in the original series. In this forced-choice recognition format, the subjects have to choose which one they have already seen. The word memory part of the test is given with identical instructions. The subject views 50 high frequency words, and then has a two-choice recognition test. Normal subjects perform very well on both parts of the test. Good age- and IQ-standardized normative data are available, including the acceptable range for a discrepancy between word and face recognition. The test is sensitive to episodic memory disorders and has the advantage of containing verbal and non-verbal tasks in the same format.

Rey Auditory Verbal Learning Test (RAVLT)

This is a verbal serial learning test using 15 common nouns. It provides a measure of immediate recall, evaluates learning over successive trials, and assesses confabulation and susceptibility to interference.

Five presentations of one list (A) are given, then one presentation of the second list (B), followed by a sixth recall trial of list A (see Box A3). The examiner reads list A at one word per second, after giving instructions along these lines: 'I am going to read you a list of words. Listen carefully, because when I stop you will have to repeat back as many as you can. It doesn't matter in what order you repeat them.'

After the first trial the examiner re-reads the same list a total of five times, using the same instructions, but emphasizing that the subject should include words recalled on previous trials. The order of the subjects' responses should be recorded each time. After Trial V of list A, the examiner reads list B and asks for recall of this list only. Finally, following the list B trial, the subject is asked to recall as many words as possible from the original list. This constitutes Trial VI.

Recall of Trial I is largely a measure of short-term (working) memory, and therefore approximates digit span to within one or two points. It varies

Box A3 Rey Auditory Verbal Learning Test (RAVLT).

List A	I	II	Trials III	IV	V	List B	Trial Recall	VI
1 Drum	–	–	–	–	–	1 Book	–	–
2 Curtain	–	–	–	–	–	2 Flower	–	–
3 Bell	–	–	–	–	–	3 Train	–	–
4 Coffee	–	–	–	–	–	4 Rug	–	–
5 School	–	–	–	–	–	5 Meadow	–	–
6 Parent	–	–	–	–	–	6 Harp	–	–
7 Moon	–	–	–	–	–	7 Salt	–	–
8 Garden	–	–	–	–	–	8 Finger	–	–
9 Hat	–	–	–	–	–	9 Apple	–	–
10 Farmer	–	–	–	–	–	10 Chimney	–	–
11 Nose	–	–	–	–	–	11 Button	–	–
12 Turkey	–	–	–	–	–	12 Key	–	–
13 Colour	–	–	–	–	–	13 Dog	–	–
14 House	–	–	–	–	–	14 Glass	–	–
15 River	–	–	–	–	–	15 Rattle	–	–
Total	–	–	–	–	–	–	–	–

according to age and education, so that elderly (>70 years) subjects recall 5 (± 1) and young professionals recall 7–8 (± 1.5). Normal subjects show considerable learning across Trials I–V, with a mean increment of 5 or 6 words above their Trial I recall, and relatively little age-variation. A drop of 3 or more words between trials V and VI of list A is regarded as abnormal. Further details are given in Lezak, Howieson and Loring's book (see Selected Further Reading).

Like the RMT, the RAVLT test is sensitive to episodic memory disorders. Patients with the amnesic syndrome show reasonable recall on Trial I, but very little learning over successive trials. They are also sensitive to the interference effects of list B, and tend to confabulate, producing items extraneous to either list.

Rey–Osterrieth Complex Figure Test (Harcourt Assessment Resources, Inc.)

The Complex Figure Test can be used to evaluate both visuo-constructional ability and visual memory. Subjects are asked to copy the figure (see Figure A7)

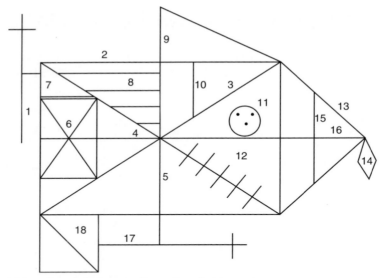

Fig. A7 Rey–Osterrieth Complex Figure Test. Scoring system.

freehand, without time restriction. A note should be made of their general approach to the task and organizational skills. Some examiners use a sequence of different coloured pencils, which they pass to the subject at 30 s intervals; but this is probably unnecessary in ordinary clinical practice. After a delay, typically 30–40 min, subjects are asked to reproduce the figure without prior warning. Some neuropsychologists also test recall after a few minutes' delay.

Copying skills are severely disrupted by right hemisphere damage, often with a tendency to neglect the left side of the figure. Patients with extensive left hemisphere lesions may also copy the figure in a disorganized, piecemeal fashion and frontal patients tend to draw impoverished figures with perseverated elements.

Recall is very poor in patients with the amnesic syndrome, and with selective right temporal lobe damage. Performance on the copy *and* recall portions of the test are extremely poor in patients with moderate-to-severe Alzheimer's disease; but recall is selectively impaired in mild disease.

As well as a qualitative assessment, the accuracy of the copied and recalled versions can be scored using the standardized scoring system shown in Box A4, which allots a maximum of two points to each of the 18 elements of the figure. Normative data are shown in Box A5.

Box A4 Scoring System for Reg-Osterrieth Figure Test

Scoring system	Score	
Units	Copy	Recall
1. Cross upper left corner, outside of rectangle		
2. Large rectangle		
3. Diagonal cross		
4. Horizontal midline of 2		
5. Vertical midline of 2		
6. Small rectangle within 2, to the left		
7. Small segment above 6		
8. Small parallel lines within 2, upper left		
9. Triangle above 2, upper right		
10. Small vertical line within 2, below 9		
11. Circle with 3 dots within 2		
12. Five parallel lines within 2 crossing 3, lower right		
13. Sides of triangle attached to 2 on right		
14. Diamond attached to 13		
15. Vertical line within triangle 13, parallel to right vertical of 2		
16. Horizontal line within 13, continuing 4 to right		
17. Cross attached to low centre		
18. Square attached to 2, lower left		
Total		

	Placed poorly	Properly placed
Correct	1	2
Distorted or incomplete	1/2	1
Absent or Not recognizable	0	0
		Max.: 36

Box A5 Rey–Osterrieth Complex Figure Test Normative Data

Normative data	Copy	30 min recall
Adults <60 years	32 ± 2	22 ± 4
Elderly subjects	28 ± 3	13 ± 4

Rivermead Behavioural Memory Test: Second Edition (RBMT-II) (Harcourt Assessment Resources, Inc.)

The RBMT was developed initially to assess memory recovery in brain-injured patients. It combines conventional tasks (for example, orientation and story recall) with more real-life tasks (for example, remembering a route and a message) that arguably correlate more closely with psychosocial competence. It is an easy-to-use measure, not requiring special professional training to administer and to score. However, it does take 20–30 min to administer. It provides an overall screening score for significant memory impairment, as well as more detailed scores for each of the subtests listed below.

1. Remembering a person's first name and surname, tested by associating the names with a face (photograph) and asking for the names when the photograph is shown again later (without warning).

2. Remembering 10 common objects (which the subject is required to name and study), and five faces. The initial stimuli (objects, faces) are represented with the same number of additional distracting objects, and the subject is required to identify the objects/faces initially seen.

3. Remembering the gist of a short prose passage, tested immediately and again after a 20 min delay.

4. Following a route around a room visiting five specified points, first immediately after being shown and then 20 min later. (A model or drawing can be used for immobile patients.) The patient is also asked to leave a message (envelope) at one point.

5. Remembering to ask for a personal belonging, which has been taken from the patient at the beginning, at the end of the test (20–30 min delay).

6. Remembering a particular question (asking about the next appointment), the question being given initially with instructions to ask it when an alarm bell rings 20 min later.

7. Ten questions to test orientation in time, place and person, and one question asking for the date.

Items scored (for RBMT screening score):

1. First name of person in photograph.
2. Second name (surname) of person in photograph.
3. Remembering hidden belonging.
4. Remembering to ask about appointment (question after alarm sounds).
5. Picture (object) recognition (selecting 10 from 20 shown).
6a. Prose recall—immediate (21 ideas).
6b. Prose recall—delayed (20 min).
7. Face recognition (recognizing five from 10 shown).
8a. Route—immediate (five places).
8b. Route—delayed (about 20 min).
9. Route—message (envelope to be left).
10. Orientation.
11. Date (correct).

Story Recall (Logical Memory)

A number of different paragraph or story recall tests have been used, all of which derive from the Logical Memory Subtest of the Wechsler Memory Scale (WMS), or are modifications of the Babcock story. In the WMS and WMS-R, two stories are used, each containing 25 elements; the score is taken as the mean of those for the two stories. It is usual to test both immediate recall and delayed recall after an interval of 30–45 min. The latter has been shown to be particularly sensitive to episodic memory disorders (for example, the amnesic syndrome, Alzheimer's disease, etc.), and to correlate well with real-life memory difficulties. A example is given in Box A6.

Subjects should be instructed as follows:

"I am going to read a short story to you now. Listen carefully because when I have finished I am going to ask you to tell me as much of the story as you can remember." After reading the story, the examiner instructs the patient "Now tell me everything you can remember." Recall is again tested after a delay of approximately 30 min, without prior warning.

A full credit is given for each element of the story recalled correctly. A half credit is given for synonyms, substitutes, or omissions of an adjective or verb that do not alter the basic idea-unit. The test is very sensitive in normal subjects to the effects of age and general intellectual ability. Box A6 gives a rough guide to the expected normal levels using this test.

Hence, a 60-year-old of high intelligence would be expected to recall more than 10 elements immediately, and to retain at least 60 per cent after a delay.

Box A6 Example of a Prose Passage and Age-related Norms for Recall

Mary /Allen / of North / Oxford, / employed / as a cook / in a college, / reported / at the police / station / that she had been held up / in Broad Street / that morning / and robbed / of £50. She had three / little children, / the rent was due, / and they had not eaten / for 24 hours. / The Officers, / touched by the woman's story, / made up a purse / for her. [Total elements = 24]

	Age (years)			
	20–39	**40–59**	**60–69**	**70–79**
Immediate recall, mean (SD)	10.0 (2.5)	8.0 (2.5)	7.5 (3.0)	6.0 (3.0)
Delayed recall as % of immediate mean (SD)	60% (20%)	55% (20%)	70% (15%)	65% (15%)

A normal seventy-year-old of low intellectual ability could recall as little as four elements initially, and retain a third after a delay.

Stroop Tests

These are based on the fact that it takes longer to call out the colour names of coloured patches than to read words, and even longer to name the colour of an ink in which a colour name is printed when the print ink is a colour different from the colour name. The latter phenomena, a markedly slowed response when a colour name is printed in ink of a different colour, is interpreted as cognitive slowing due to response conflict or a failure of selective attention.

A great number of versions of this test have been published which vary in the number of trials and items. Some formats use only two trials: one in which reading focuses on colour words printed in ink of different colours and the other requiring naming of the colour patches. This includes the popular Dodrill version recommended by Lezak, Howieson and Loring in *Neuropsychological Assessment* (4th edition). Versions also vary in the number of items in the trial and the number of colours used. A version of the Stroop is included in the D-KEFS test (see p. 227). The Dodrill version consists of a single sheet containing 176 colour names randomly printed in one of four colours (red, orange, green, blue). In part I, the subject reads the printed word names and in part II the subject reports the colour in which each word is printed (see Figure A8). A maximum of 300 s are allowed for part I and 600 s for part II. Normal controls typically complete part I

RED	GREEN	BLUE	BLACK
BLUE	PINK	RED	BLACK
YELLOW	BLACK	ORANGE	BLUE
RED	GREEN	RED	ORANGE
GRAY	YELLOW	GREEN	GREEN
BROWN	PINK	BLUE	BLACK
BLUE	BROWN	YELLOW	BLUE
RED	ORANGE	GREEN	RED
GREEN	PINK	BLACK	YELLOW

Fig. A8 Example of Stroop Test. See colour plate section.

in around 90 ± 20 s and part II in 230 ± 70 s. The key score is the difference between parts II and I, which is markedly prolonged in patients with a variety of brain pathologies including epilepsy and early-stage Alzheimer's disease.

Test for the Reception of Grammar (TROG-II) (Harcourt Assessment Resources, Inc.)

This test was developed by Bishop for use in children with developmental language disorders but is very useful in the neuropsychological population. It is a sentence–picture matching test that uses low-level vocabulary items (such as horse, boy, flower) and is cleverly designed to test syntactic comprehension of increasing complexity. Subjects are presented with a page comprising four pictures and are asked to choose the picture which matches the word, or sentence, spoken by the examiner. The early blocks are designed to check comprehension of the vocabulary items. Subsequent blocks increase in complexity such that later trials probe constructions such as embedded clauses and reversible structures. The total possible score is 80. Most normal adults obtain scores in the high 70s, failing occasional items in later complex blocks. By contrast, patients with deficits in sentence comprehension as a result of stroke or neurodegeneration have great difficulty and begin to fail on earlier items in the test.

The Token Test (Pro-ed Publications, Inc.)

The Token Test is a sensitive and reliable measure of auditory comprehension in aphasic stroke patients, although its value in other language-disordered patients is less clear. It is easy to administer and score, and the material needed can be readily made. Twenty 'tokens' cut from cardboard, plastic or wood are used. They come in two sizes: big and small; two shapes: circles and squares; and five colours. The original version consisted of 62 commands, graded from the very simple (for example, "Touch the red circle and touch the small green square") to syntactically complex commands (for example, "Put the red circle on the green square" and "Pick up all the squares except the yellow one").

A shortened version, consisting of 36 commands, has been widely used. Educationally standardized normative data are available.

Trail Making Test

This is a quick and easily administered test of visuo-motor tracking, and of conceptualization and mental 'set shifting'. A version of the trails is included in the D-KEFS battery (see p. 227). It is given in two parts (A and B). Part A consists of a series of circles enclosing numbers from 1 to 25, scattered at random on the page. The subject's task is to join the circles in numerical order as quickly as possible. Part B has both numbers and letters arrayed in the random order. The subject must alternate between numbers and letters: 1 to A to 2 to B to 3 to C, and so on to 13 (see Figure A9).

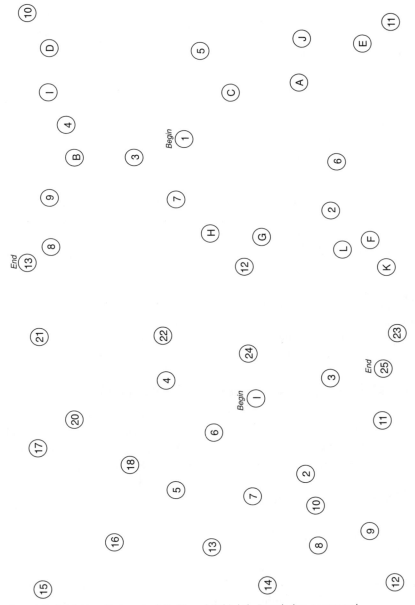

Fig. A9 Trail Making Test parts A (left) and B (right). Permission requested.

Box A7 Age-adjusted upper limits (10th + 25th percentiles) for normality (in seconds) on the Trail Making Test

	Age (years)				
	20–39	40–49	50–59	60–69	70–79
Part A					
10%	42	45	49	67	105
25%	50	59	67	104	168
Part B					
10%	95	100	135	172	292
25%	130	150	177	282	450

Various administration and scoring procedures have been used; but it is usual to point out errors as they occur, to allow self-correction, and to score only in terms of time to complete.

In common with any test that depends upon response-speed, performance on trail making depends markedly on age. Approximate age-adjusted upper limits for normality in seconds are given in Box A7.

Impaired performance on either part of the test can result from motor slowing, incoordination, visual scanning difficulties, poor motivation, or frontal executive problems. Patients with frontal lobe dysfunction perform disproportionately badly on Part B.

Verbal Fluency Tests: Letter and Category Fluency

Verbal fluency, sometimes referred to as controlled oral word-association, is a very useful bedside test which is sensitive to frontal 'executive' dysfunction and subtle degrees of semantic memory impairment. A number of versions based on letter and semantic category have been used. The most extensive experience is of 'FAS' for letter fluency, and the category 'animals'.

FAS: Subjects are asked to list as many words as possible beginning with each of the three letters in turn. One minute is allowed per letter. Subjects are told beforehand that proper nouns (personal and place names) and repetitions of words with different suffixes (find, finder, finding, etc.) are not acceptable.

Animals: Subjects are asked to list as many animals as possible in 1 min. If this test is given immediately after letter fluency, it is important to point out that the animal names can begin with any letter.

Scores for the total responses, the number of perseverative errors, and other (intrusive) errors can be obtained. For FAS, it is usual to summate across the three letters. Normal subjects should not perseverate or lose set (i.e. revert to a prior letter). Performance depends on age and education. Young professionals should produce in excess of 45 words for FAS and a total of 30 or below is abnormal. The lowest acceptable total for elderly subjects of low educational attainment is around 25 words. Category fluency is usually superior to letter fluency. For the category animals, normal subjects usually produce 20 exemplars. The lower limit of acceptability ranges from 12 to 15, again depending on age and education.

The Visual Object and Space Perception Battery (VOSP) (Harcourt Assessment Resources, Inc.)

This battery of eight visuo-perceptual tests was recently developed, validated and standardized by Warrington and James. Each subset was developed to focus on one component of visual perception, while minimizing the contribution of other cognitive skills. Most of the tasks are based on prior experimental studies performed by the authors. All are sensitive to right hemisphere damage, and normative values are included with the battery.

An initial simple figure–ground discrimination test screens out patients with severe visual handicap. The battery proper consists of four tests of object recognition and four tests of space perception.

Object Recognition

1. *Incomplete letters* consists of letters fragmented by varying degrees of masking. A simple version of this is included in the ACE-R.

2. *Silhouettes* assesses the subject's ability to recognize common objects photographed from an unusual view.

3. *Object decision* contains arrays of four silhouettes: one real object and three nonsense shapes. The task is to select the real object (see Figure A10).

4. *Progressive silhouettes* consists of objects photographed from progressively less rotated viewpoints. The subject is required to identify the object as soon as possible.

Space Perception

5. *Dot counting* consists of arrays of five to eight black dots on white cards, which the subject is asked to count. Four examples based on this task are included in the ACE-R.

A

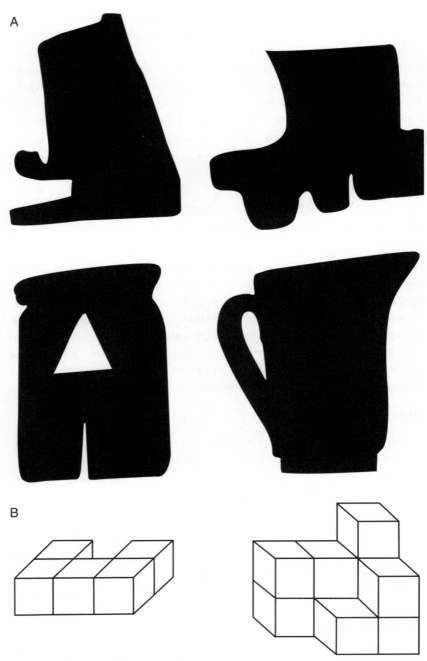

B

Fig. A10 Examples of the object decision (A) and cube analysis (B) subtests of the Visual Object and Space Perception Battery. Copyright © 1991 by Elizabeth K. Warrington and Merle James. Reproduced with permission of Harcourt Assessment, Inc.

6. *Position discrimination* consists of two adjacent squares: one has a dot in the centre, and in the other it is off-centre. The subject has to choose the square with the centrally placed dot.

7. *Number location* is similar to the former test, but in this test one square contains randomly arranged numbers and the other a single black dot corresponding in position to one of the numbers. The task is to select the number that matches the position of the dot.

8. *Cube analysis* tests the ability of subjects to judge the number of bricks present in a three-dimensional arrangement of square blocks of increasing complexity (see Figure A10).

Wechsler Adult Intelligence Scale (WAIS-R and WAIS-III) (Harcourt Assessment Resources, Inc.)

The WAIS-R (1981) and the most recently updated version, the WAIS-III (1997), remain the most widely used test batteries for evaluating general intellectual and neuropsychological ability. For most clinical neuropsychologists, they form the cornerstone of cognitive assessment. A great strength of the WAIS batteries lies in their comprehensive standardization. The WAIS-R included data on 1880 subjects aged 16–87 years and the WAIS-III 2450 subjects aged 16–89 years. A full description of the WAIS-III is beyond the scope of this book. Its administration and scoring are relatively complex and demand formal training. Interpretation of the results depends upon considerable experience. The subject's behaviour, general approach to testing, and types of errors produced form an important part of the evaluation.

The WAIS-R consists of 11 subtests (six verbal and five performance), to which have been added three new tests—Letter-Number Sequencing, Symbol Search and Matrix Reasoning—for the WAIS-III. By summating the subtest scores and adjusting for age, Verbal, Performance and Full Scale IQ scores can be derived. An average person should obtain a score of 100 for each, one standard deviation being 15 points. In neuropsychological practice, however, the pattern of individual subtest scores is usually more informative than the overall IQ. Each subtest yields a raw score, which can be converted into a scaled score. An average subject should obtain a scaled score of 10, with the standard deviation being 3 points. But the 'normal' range varies considerably with age; the performance subtests are particularly vulnerable to the effects of ageing. By correcting for age, **age-scaled scores** for each subtest can be derived.

In addition to the full WAIS-III, there is the new Wechsler Abbreviated Scale of Intelligence (WASI-1999) designed to be a short form with parallel tests which yields Full Scale, Verbal and Performance IQ scores. The four tests in the battery are Vocabulary, Similarities, Block Design and Matrix Reasoning. Each test is similar in form and content to its WAIS-III counterpart but contains different stimuli.

The correlation between specific subtests and individual cognitive functions, and hence pathologies, is relatively poor, because many of the subtests tap several cognitive abilities simultaneously. For instance, Picture Arrangement is dependent upon visuo-perceptual and planning abilities; therefore it is susceptible to both right hemisphere and frontal lobe damage.

A full account of the tests and their interpretation can be found in *Neuropsychological Assessment* (3rd edition) by Lezak, Howieson and Loring (see 'Selected further reading'). A brief description of each of the WAIS subtests is included here to aid clinicians with little or no experience of the test battery.

Verbal scales subtests

1. *Information* is a test of general knowledge that consists of 29 questions arranged in order of difficulty from 'How many months are there in a year?' and 'What is a thermometer?' to 'How many Members of Parliament are there in the House of Commons?' and 'Who wrote *Faust*?'

2. *Comprehension* includes 16 open-ended questions that test common sense, judgement, and practical reasoning. Examples are 'Why do people have to register their marriage?' and 'Why do people who are born deaf have difficulty learning to talk?'

3. *Arithmetic* contains 14 tests of mental arithmetic of increasing complexity, such as 'How much is £4 and £5?' and 'How many hours would it take to walk 24 miles at a rate of 3 miles per hour?'

4. *Similarities* is a test of verbal concept-formation in which the subject must explain what a pair of words has in common. The 14 word-pairs range in difficulty from 'orange/banana' and 'coat/dress' to 'poem/statue' and 'praise/punishment'.

5. *Digit span* tests the ability of subjects to repeat sequences of digits of increasing length first in the same order (digits forward) and then in reverse order (digits backwards). It is also included in the Wechsler Memory Scale. Further details can be found on p. 254.

6. *Vocabulary* consists of 35 words that the subject is asked to define. It starts with extremely common words, such as 'bed' and 'winter', and concludes with the infrequent words 'encumber', 'audacious', and 'tirade'.

Performance scale subtests

Four of the five subtests require motor responses—one writing and three manipulating material. All of them are time-limited, and there are extra credits for rapid completion on several.

1. *Digit–symbol substitution* consists of four rows of blank squares each paired with a randomly assigned number from 1 to 9. Above the array is a key that pairs each number with a nonsense symbol. The subject's task is to fill as many blank squares as possible in 90 s using the digit–symbol key above.

2. *Picture completion* has 20 incomplete pictures of familiar objects or scenes, with instructions to report which important part is missing. Examples include a knobless door, spectacles without the bridge section, and a violin with three pegs.

3. *Block design* is a constructional test in which the subject has to make various patterns using red and white blocks. The subject first copies simple four-block designs made by the examiner, and then copies increasingly complex designs of up to nine blocks from examples printed on small cards.

4. *Picture arrangement* contains 10 sets of cartoon pictures that make up stories. The subject is presented with each set in a scrambled order, and is asked to rearrange them to make the most sensible story in as short a time as possible.

5. *Object assembly* consists of four cut-up jigsaw-like cardboard figures of familiar objects (a manikin, a face in profile, a hand, and an elephant). The subject is presented with each in turn in a scrambled array, and is asked to reassemble the figure as quickly as possible.

Additional tests in WAIS-III

1. *Matrix Reasoning.* This has the same basic features as Raven's Progressive Matrices in that it presents a series of increasingly difficult visual pattern completion and analogy problems.

2. *Letter–Number Sequencing.* Subjects hear lists of randomized numbers and letters (in alternating order) of increasing length (from two to eight units). Subjects are asked to repeat numbers and letters from the lowest in each series, and numbers always first. For example, in hearing "6–F–2–B", the subject should respond "2–6–B–F". The span is increased until the subject fails all three items at one length.

3. *Symbol Search.* This subtest is very similar to Digit Symbol Substitution.

Wechsler Memory Scale (WMS) and Wechsler Memory Scale—Revised (WMS-R) (Harcourt Assessment Resources, Inc.)

The WMS was, for many years, the standard tool for the assessment of suspected memory disorders. It consisted of six subtests measuring orientation, mental control (attention), digit span, logical memory (story recall), verbal paired associate learning, and visual reproduction of geometrical figures. From these six subtests, a general Memory Quotient (MQ) could be obtained. The MQ was based on the sum of the raw scores. This total raw score was transformed with suitable age-adjustment to the MQ in such a way that it approximated to the Full Scale IQ of the WAIS. Thus an average person should obtain a Full Scale IQ of 100 and an MQ of 100, with the standard deviation of each being 15 points. A discrepancy between IQ and MQ of more than 15 points therefore indicates significant memory impairment. The major criticism of the WMS has been the bias towards verbal memory, the absence of delayed recall conditions for any of the subtests, and inclusion in the MQ score of subtests more dependent upon attentional processes (mental control and orientation) than upon memory *per se*.

The WMS-R is a considerable improvement. It incorporates two new visual memory tests (figural memory and visual paired associates), a new visual counterpart of digit span (visual memory span), a number of administration changes and, most importantly, delayed recall conditions for two of the verbal and two of the visual memory tests. As well as producing raw scores for each of the subtests, separate age-adjusted indices can now be obtained for Verbal, Visual, and General Memory, Attention/Concentration, and Delayed Recall. The memory indices are free from the contaminating effects of attentional deficits. Extensive normative data are accruing, as well as data on patients with common cognitive disorders.

The WMS and WMS-R are not appropriate tests for use at the bedside or in the clinic. Their administration requires expertise, and the scoring system is fairly complex. The digit span and logical memory subtests are the most easily adaptable. These provide good measures of attention and of verbal episodic memory, respectively. Everyday versions of these two subtests are described elsewhere (see pp. 227 and 241). The remainder of the subtests are described below, to familiarize clinicians with their content, and thus to aid the interpretation of neuropsychological reports.

1. *Information and orientation* contains 14 standard time, place and person orientation items, plus general information questions (mother's maiden name, President of the USA, etc.).

2. *Mental control* consists of rapid serial counting (20 to 1), alphabet recitation, and serial addition (1, 4, 7, etc.).

3. *Digit span* requires subjects to repeat in forward and reverse order strings of digits of increasing length.

4. *Logical memory* consists of two stories, each of 25 elements, which the subject is asked to recall immediately after hearing and again after a 30 min delay.

5. *Verbal paired associates* tests subjects' ability to make word associations. The subject is read a group of eight word-pairs; half are easy to associate (for example metal–iron, baby–cries) and half are hard to associate (crush–dark, obey–inch). Subjects are then read the first word of the pair and asked to supply the second word. Up to six trials are given of the same list, but with the word-pairs arranged in different orders. After a delay, the recall is again rested, without prior warning.

6. *Visual memory span* is analogous to digit span, and consists of 'tapping forwards' and 'tapping backwards'. The subject is presented with an array of red squares randomly arranged on a card. On 'tapping forwards', the subject watches the examiner touch red squares in sequences of increasing length, and after each sequence is asked to repeat the sequence from memory. On 'tapping backwards', the subject again watches the examiner touch sequences of increasing length, and is asked to repeat the performance in reverse order.

7. *Visual reproduction* requires the subject to reproduce from memory four geometrical designs, each shown for 10 s. After a delay of 30 min, the subject is again asked to draw the figures without prior warning.

8. *Figural memory* is a short-term visual memory test in which the subjects look at abstract designs (shaded block drawings) for 5 s; immediately afterwards they are asked to choose, from three alternatives, which design they have just seen.

9. *Visual paired associates* is analogous to the verbal paired associates test. The subject is shown six abstract line-drawings, each paired with a different colour, and is then shown the drawings alone, and is asked to recall the colour associated with each figure.

Wechsler Memory Scale-III (WMS-III) (Harcourt Assessment Resources, Inc.)

The WMS-III published in 1997 represents the latest attempt to present a comprehensive approach to memory assessment. It contains an even larger number of tests than the WMS-R, considerably lengthening the battery. The core battery consists of six tests, three of which appeared in the WMS-R to calculate various memory indices. Five tests are optional, four of which appeared in a slightly different form in the previous edition.

The WMS-R tests included, with slight alterations, are Logical Memory, Verbal Paired Associates and Spatial Span. The new WMS-III core battery tests are: Letter–Number Sequencing, Faces and Family Pictures. Information and Orientation, Mental Control, Digit Span and Visual Reproduction are now classified as optional tests along with a newly developed verbal test, named Word-Lists. The normative data for the WMS-III have been considerably extended to include 1250 subjects with the highest age-bracket range now being 85–95 years.

The WMS-III tests generate eight primary memory indices: Auditory Immediate, Visual Immediate, Combined Immediate Memory, Auditory Delayed, Visual Delayed, Auditory Recognition Delayed, General Memory Delayed and Working Memory.

The newer tests are described briefly below.

1. *Letter–number sequencing*. This test is also included in the WAIS-R.

2. *The faces test* has both immediate and delayed components and is a recognition task in which 24 faces are shown, one at a time, for approximately 2 s each. Immediate and delayed recognition are tested using a yes–no format in which targets are interspersed with an equal number of foils.

3. *Family pictures* is designed to measure complex, meaningful, visually presented information. Four pictures are shown to the subject for 10 s each. Memory is tested using free recall for four persons from a family of seven (e.g. mother, father, grandmother, son, dog, etc.), what they are doing in the picture and their location on a 2 × 2 grid. Immediate and delayed recall are obtained.

4. *Word-list* is a word-learning task containing 12 words that have no semantic association presented over four trials, followed by a single trial of a second, interference list. Then, without further additional presentation, recall of the first list is required. Two delayed trials follow: free recall, and yes–no recognition in which the examiner reads the 12 words interspersed among 12 foils.

The WMS-III is obviously a sophisticated memory battery that requires training. At the time of writing this book, evidence on its application in neuropsychology has been limited but it is likely that neuropsychologists will adopt the core tasks.

RED	GREEN	BLUE	BLACK
BLUE	PINK	RED	BLACK
YELLOW	BLACK	ORANGE	BLUE
RED	GREEN	RED	ORANGE
GRAY	YELLOW	GREEN	GREEN
BROWN	PINK	BLUE	BLACK
BLUE	BROWN	YELLOW	BLUE
RED	ORANGE	GREEN	RED
GREEN	PINK	BLACK	YELLOW

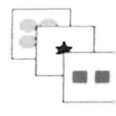

Western Aphasia Battery (WAB) (Harcourt Assessment Resources, Inc.)

This instrument is similar to the longer and older Boston Diagnostic Aphasia Examination. It comprises four oral language subtests—spontaneous speech, auditory comprehension, repetition and naming—which together yield five scores based on either a rating scale or conversion of summed item correct scores to a scale of 10. Each score can therefore be charted on a 10-point scale together to produce a profile of performance. An **Aphasia Quotient** can be calculated by multiplying each of the five scaled scores by two and summing. Normal (i.e. perfect) performance is set at 100. The profile of performance can be used to determine the patient's diagnostic subtype according to classic descriptions of classic aphasia syndromes. In addition, tests of reading, writing, arithmetic, gestural praxis, construction and reasoning are included to provide a comprehensive survey of communication abilities and related functions. The language portion of the test takes 1½ h to complete. As well as in patients with post-stroke aphasia, WAB data have been published in patients with Alzheimer's disease, progressive aphasia and vascular dementia.

The Wisconsin Card Sorting Test (WCST) (Harcourt Assessment Resources, Inc.)

This widely used test was designed to study 'abstract behaviour' and 'set-shifting ability'. It is sensitive to frontal lobe damage, particularly that involving the left dorsolateral area, and is failed by patients with dementing illnesses, particularly those of the subcortical type, but can be impaired in subjects with lesions elsewhere. The subject is given a pack of 64 cards on which are printed one to four symbols (triangle, star, cross, or circle) in one of four colours (see Figure A11). The subjects' task is to place them, one by one, under four stimulus cards consisting of: one red triangle, two green circles, three yellow squares, and four blue stars, according to a principle that the patient must deduce from the examiner's responses. The examiner tells the subject if the choice was "right" or "wrong". For instance, if the principle is colour, the correct placement of the red card is under the red triangle, regardless of form of symbol or number. After 10 correct sorts, the examiner shifts the principle indicating the shift only in the changed pattern of "right" or "wrong" responses. The test begins with colour, then shifts to form, and then to number, before returning again to colour and so on. The most widely used scores are for number of categories achieved (maximum 6) and number of perseverative errors. Perseverative errors occur when the subject continues to sort according to a previously successful principle

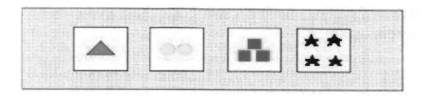

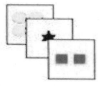

Fig. A11 Wisconsin Card Sorting Test. Reproduced with special permission of the Publisher, Psychological Assessment Resources, Inc., from the Wisconsin Card Sorting Test by David A. Grant and Esta A. Berg. Copyright 1981, 1993 by PAR, Inc. See colour plate section.

or, in the first series, when the subject persists in sorting on the basis of an initial erroneous guess.

The Modified Card Sorting Test (MCST) eliminates from the pack all cards that share more than one attribute with the stimulus card and the pack comprises only 48 cards. Whichever sorting dimension is chosen first is designated correct and more explicit shifting instructions are given. It is otherwise similar to the longer version. Further details are given in *Neuropsychological Assessment* (4th edition) by Lezak, Howieson and Loring (see 'Selected further reading').

Addresses of Publishers

BrainMetric
52–13 Revere Rd
Drexel Hill
PA 19026
USA
www.brainmetric.com

Cambridge Cognition Ltd
Tunbridge Court
Tunbridge Lane
Bottisham

Cambridge CB25 9TU
UK
www.cantab.com
Harcourt Assessment, Inc.
Halley Court
Jordan Hill
Oxford OX2 8EJ
UK
www.harcourt-uk.com

NFER—Nelson
Windsor
Berks SL4 1BU
UK
www.nfer-nelson.co.uk

Pro-ed Publications, Inc.
8700 Shoal Creek Boulevard
Austin
TX 78751-6897
USA
www.proedinc.com

Psychological Assessment Resources, Inc. (PAR)
16204 N
Florida Avenue
Lutz
FL 33549
USA
www.parinc.com

Selected Further Reading

Andrews, D. G. (2001). *Neuropsychology from Theory to Practice.* Psychology Press, Hove, UK.

Baddeley, A. D. (1997). *Human Memory: Theory and Practice* (revised edition). Alleyn & Bacon, London, UK.

Bak, T. H., Caine, D., Hearn, V. C., & Hodges, J. R. (2006). Visuospatial functions in atypical parkinsonian syndromes. *Journal of Neurology, Neurosurgery and Psychiatry,* 77, 454–456.

Berrios, G. E., Hodges, J. R. (eds) (2000). *Memory Disorders in Psychiatric Practice.* Cambridge University Press, Cambridge, UK.

Burns, A., O'Brien, J., Ames, D. (eds) (1993). *Dementia* (3rd edition). Hodder Arnold, London, UK.

Cummings, J. L. (ed.) (2003). *The Neuropsychiatry of Alzheimer's Disease and Related Disorders.* Martin Dunitz, London, UK.

D'Esposito, M. (ed.) (2003). *Neurological Foundations of Cognitive Neuroscience.* MIT Press, Cambridge, Massachusetts, USA.

Dudas, R. B., Berrios, G. E., & Hodges, J. R. (2005). The Addenbrooke's Cognitive Examination (ACE) in the Differential Diagnosis of Early Organic Dementias from Affective disorder. *American Journal of Geriatric Psychiatry,* 13, 218–226.

Ellis, A. W., Young, A. W. (1988). *Human Cognitive Neuropsychology.* Lawrence Erlbaum, Hove and London, UK.

Feinberg, T., Farah, M. (1997). *Behavioural Neurology and Neuropsychology.* McGraw-Hill, New York, USA.

Halligan, P. W., Kischka, U., Marshall, J. C. (2003). *Handbook of Clinical Neuropsychology.* Oxford University Press, Oxford, UK.

Heilman, K. M. and Valenstein, E. (2003). *Clinical Neuropsychology* (4th edition). Oxford University Press, New York, USA.

Hodges, J. R. (1991). *Transient Amnesia: Clinical and Neuropsychological Aspects.* W. B. Saunders, London, UK.

Hodges, J. R. (ed.) (2001). *Early-onset Dementia: A Multidisciplinary Approach.* Oxford University Press, Oxford, UK.

Hodges, J. R. (ed.) (2007). *Frontotemporal Dementia Syndromes.* Cambridge University Press, Cambridge, UK.

Lezak, M. D., Howieson, D. B., Loring, D. W. (2004). *Neuropsychological Assessment* (4th edition). Oxford University Press, New York, USA.

Lipowski, Z. T. (1990). *Delirium: Acute Confusional States.* Oxford University Press, New York, USA.

Lishman, W. A. (1998). *Organic Psychiatry: The Psychological Consequences of Cerebral Disorder* (3rd edition). Blackwell Scientific, Oxford, UK.

Luria, A. R. (1966). *Higher Cortical Function in Man.* Tavistock, London, UK.

Mathuranath, P. S., Nestor, P., Berrios, G. E., Rakowicz, W., & Hodges, J. R. (2000). A brief cognitive test battery to differentiate Alzheimer's disease and frontotemporal dementia. *Neurology*, 55, 1613–1620.

McCarthy, R. A., Warrington, E. K. (1990). *Cognitive Neuropsychology: A Clinical Introduction*. Academic Press, San Diego, UK.

Mesulam, M. M. (ed.) (1985). *Principles of Behavioural and Cognitive Neurology* (2nd edition). Oxford University Press, New York, USA.

Mioshi, E., Dawson, K., Mitchell, J., Arnold, R., Hodges, J. R., (2006). The Addenbrooke's Cognitive Examination Revised (ACE-R): a brief cognitive test battery for dementia screening. *International Journal of Geriatric Psychiatry*, 21, 1078–1085.

Morris, R. G., Becker, J. T. (eds) (2004). *Cognitive Neuropsychology of Alzheimer's Disease*. Oxford University Press, Oxford, UK.

Petersen, R. C. (ed.) (2003). *Mild Cognitive Impairment*. Oxford University Press, New York, USA.

Rizzo, M., Eslinger, P. J. (2004). *Behavioural Neurology and Neuropsychology*. W. B. Saunders, Philadelphia, USA.

Shallice, T. (1990). *From Neuropsychology to Mental Structure*. Cambridge University Press, Cambridge, UK.

Squire, L. R. (1987). *Memory and Brain*. Oxford University Press, New York, USA.

Stuss, D. T., Benson, D. F. (1986). *The Frontal Lobes*. Lippincott, Williams & Wilkins, Baltimore, USA.

Tulving, E., Craik, F. (eds) (2000). *Oxford Handbook of Memory*. Oxford University Press, Oxford, New York, USA.

Walsh, K. W., Darby, D. (1999). *Neuropsychology: A Clinical Approach* (4th edition). Churchill Livingstone, Edinburgh, UK.

Index